Neuro-Ophthalmology Review Manual

—Second Edition—

Frank J. Bajandas, MD
Lanning B. Kline, MD

SLACK Incorporated, 6900 Grove Road, Thorofare, New Jersey 08086

Copyright © 1987 by SLACK Incorporated

Printed in the United States of America

Library of Congress Catalog Card Number: 86-42869

ISBN: 0-943432-96-0

Published by: SLACK Incorporated
6900 Grove Rd.
Thorofare, NJ 08086

Last digit is print number: 10   9   8   7   6   5   4   3   2   1

Dedication to First Edition

Gentler the Path with Familiar Footsteps to Follow
This Manual is Dedicated to
ROBERT B. DAROFF, M.D.
JOEL S. GLASER, M.D.
J. LAWTON SMITH, M.D.

Introduction to First Edition

This manual was to simply be a handy, readable compendium of the "no-nonsense" neuro-ophthalmology that neurologists, neurosurgeons, and ophthalmologists need in the ritual of preparing for Board exams. The good news is that the same material represents the clinical principles used in my everyday neuro-ophthalmology practice.

The bulk of the "brute-memory" material can be boiled down to eight diagrams.* If you can reproduce these eight diagrams, and, in turn, recall the significance of their components, you will be readily reminded of the organization of each theme and of the anatomico-physiological and pathological concepts that form the basis of clinical neuro-opthalmology.

*Fig 1-4, 1-6, 2-10, 2-11, 3-7, 3-8, 4-3, 9-1.

Introduction to Second Edition

Frank Bajandas' great abilities as a teacher were clearly demonstrated in the first edition, "Neuro-Ophthalmology Board Review Manual." He was able to organize, synthesize, and communicate the core subject material of neuro-ophthalmology in 11 chapters comprising 141 pages. While initially intended as a study guide for residents and practitioners preparing for "the Boards," this manual has become widely used by residents and fellows at all levels of training, as well as a handy reference for busy clinicians.

The revision of this teaching manual was done to update and modestly expand the material covered. The concise style and schematic illustrations have been retained. Because of the widened appeal of this book, "Board" has been deleted from the title.

My thanks go to Dr. P.S. O'Connor who contributed two chapters and critically reviewed many others. Amy Collins both revised and created many illustrations. Kathy Fleck typed the manuscript.

My family deserves special mention. Ricki, Aaron, and Evie helped me tremendously with two contributions: love and support.

Finally, I must thank Frank Bajandas, who died tragically in an automobile accident. He laid the groundwork upon which to revise and expand. I hope he would be pleased with my efforts.

Table of Contents

Frank J. Bajandas, M.D.

Associate Clinical Professor
Department of Ophthalmology
University of Texas Health Science Center
San Antonio, Texas

Lanning B. Kline, M.D.

Associate Clinical Professor
Departments of Ophthalmology, Neurology, Neurosurgery
Eye Foundation Hospital
University of Alabama School of Medicine
Birmingham, Alabama

Visual Fields

A. Traquair's Definition of the Visual Field
   Island of vision in sea of blindness (Fig. 1-1). The peak of the island represents the point of highest acuity, the fovea, while the "bottomless pit" represents the blind spot, the optic disc

B. Visual Field Testing
   1. Stimuli: testing the island of vision at various levels requires targets that vary in
      a. size
      b. intensity
      c. color
   2. Field testing methods (Fig. 1-2)
      a. Kinetic: mapping the contours of the island at different levels, resulting in one isopter for each level tested
      b. Static: vertical contours of the island along a selected meridian

C. For clinical testing the visual field can be divided into two areas (Fig. 1-3)
   1. Central: 30° radius
   2. Peripheral: beyond 30°

D. Central Visual Field
   1. Can be examined with Amsler grid, confrontation techniques, tangent screen, and bowl perimeter
   2. Confrontation techniques—see Chapter 15
   3. Amsler grid—useful in detecting subtle, central, and paracentral scotomas. When held at one-third of a meter from the patient, each square subtends one degree of visual field
   4. Tangent screen (campimetry) is excellent method to examine central field. Easier to pick up central defects with tangent screen vs. bowl perimeter. Scotomas will be three times as large at 1 meter with tangent screen as on the perimeter test surface, which is only one-third meter from patient
   5. Tangent screen not useful for testing beyond 30° because of diminishing stimulus value of test-object on flat testing surface
   6. Bowl perimeter (e.g. Goldmann) can also be used to test central 30°

E. Peripheral Visual Field
   1. Requires testing with bowl perimeter

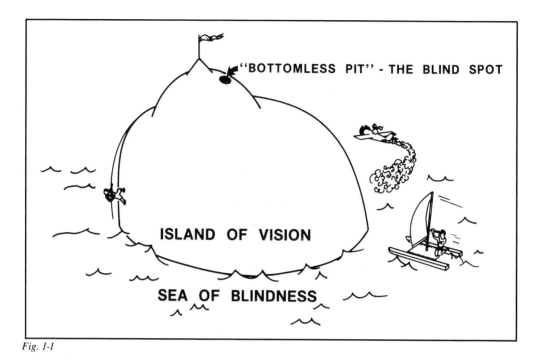

Fig. 1-1

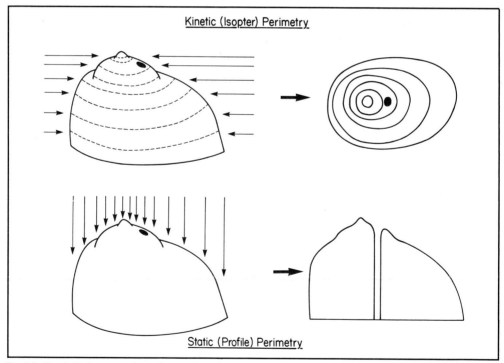

Fig. 1-2. Kinetic Perimetry: each set of target size-color-intensity and background illumination determines a different level of the island being tested, and results in a different oval-shaped cross-section or isopter; note the six isopters at right, the result of testing six levels of the island Static Perimetry: the target is held stationary at different points along the selected meridian; the intensity of the target is slowly increased until it is defected by the patient; the intensity required determines the upper level (i.e., the greatest sensitivity) of the island at this point.

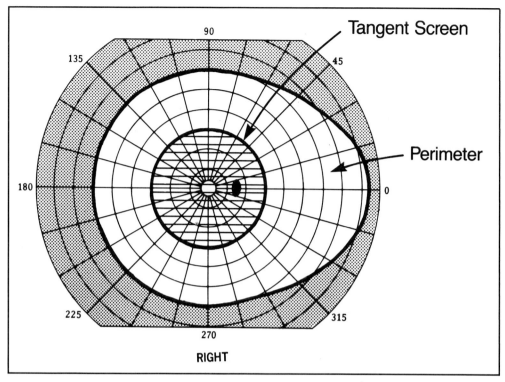

Fig. 1-3. Central visual field (30-degree radius) can be tested with tangent screen, while entire field can be tested with perimeter.

    2. Particularly helpful in detecting
       a. ring scotoma (retinitis pigmentosa)
       b. nasal step (glaucoma)
       c. temporal crescent (occipital lobe)

F. Anatomy of the Visual Pathways (Fig. 1-4)

    1. The visual field and the retina have an inverted and reversed relationship. Relative to the point of fixation, the upper visual field falls on inferior retina (below the fovea), lower visual field on superior retina, nasal visual field on temporal retina, and temporal visual field on nasal retina

    2. Nasal fibers of ipsilateral eye cross in chiasm, join uncrossed temporal fibers of contralateral eye . . . optic tract . . . synapse in lateral geniculate body . . . optic radiation . . . terminate in visual cortex (area 17) of occipital lobe

    3. Lower retinal fibers and their projections lie in the lateral portion of the optic tract, and ultimately terminate in the inferior striate cortex, on the lower bank of the calcarine fissure. Upper retinal fibers project through the medial optic tract and ultimately terminate in the superior striate cortex

    4. Inferonasal retinal fibers decussate in the chiasm, travel anteriorly in the contralateral optic nerve, before passing into the optic tract. They form the knee of von Wilbrand

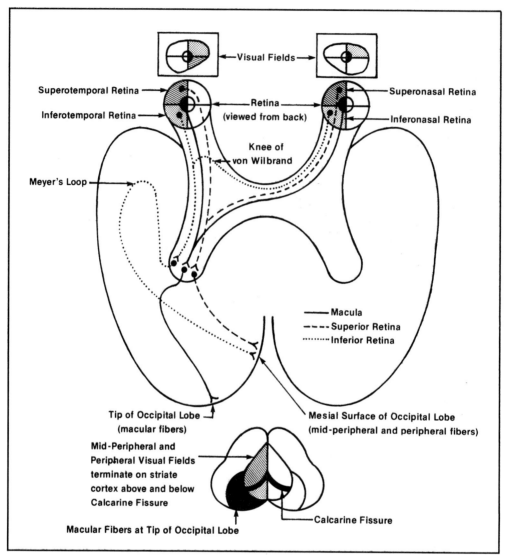

Fig. 1-4. Anatomy of the visual pathways.

G. Interpretation of Visual Field Defects
TEN KEY POINTS TO REMEMBER

1. Optic nerve-type field defects
2. "Rules of the road" for the optic chiasm
3. Optic tract—lateral geniculate body defects
4. Superior-inferior separation of the temporal lobe
5. Superior-inferior separation of the parietal lobe
6. Central homonymous hemianopia
7. Macular sparing
8. Congruity

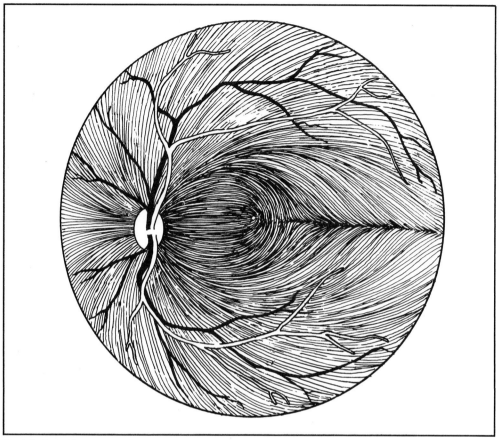

Fig. 1-5. Nerve fiber pattern of retina.

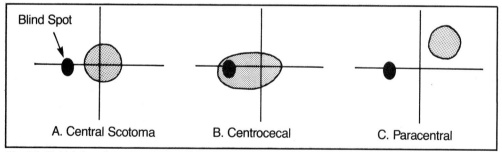

Blind Spot

A. Central Scotoma   B. Centrocecal   C. Paracentral

Fig. 1-6. Field defects due to interruption of the papillomacular bundle.

9. Optokinetic nystagmus
10. Temporal crescents
1. Optic Nerve-Type Field Defects
    a. Retinal nerve fibers enter the optic discs in a specific manner (Fig. 1-5)
    b. Nerve fiber bundle (NFB) defects are of three main types
        1) Papillomacular bundle: macular fibers that enter the temporal aspect of

5

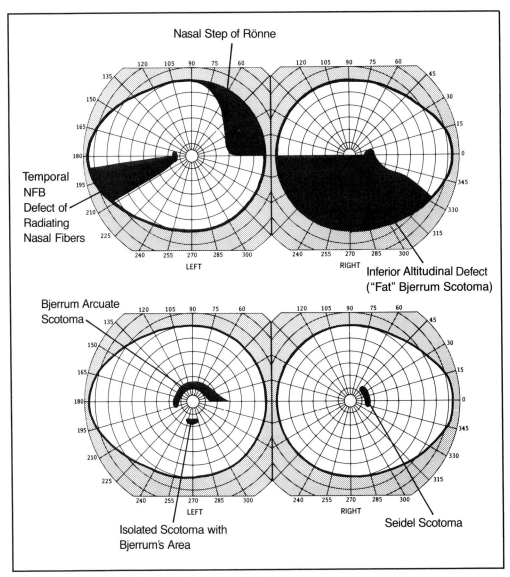

Fig. 1-7. Composite diagram depicting different types of field defects.

the disc. A defect in this bundle of nerve fibers results in one of the following

a) Central scotoma (Fig. 1-6)—a defect covering central fixation

b) Centrocecal scotoma (Fig. 1-6)—a central scotoma connected to the blind spot (the cecum)

c) Paracentral scotoma (Fig. 1-6)—a defect of some of the fibers of the papillomacular bundle, lying next to, but not involving central fixation

2) Arcuate nerve fiber bundle: fibers from the retina temporal to the disc,

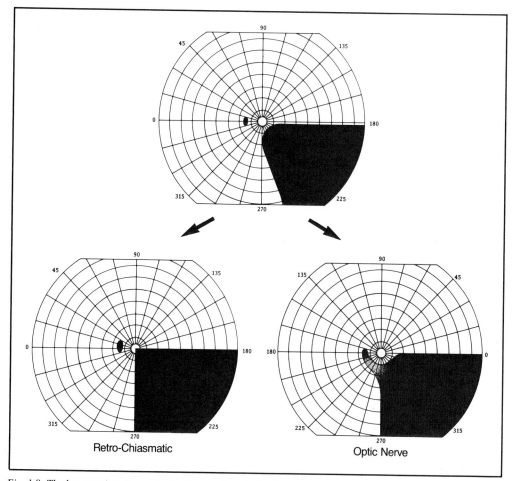

Fig. 1-8. The key question, in a patient with a quadrantic visual-field-defect: does the field defect go to fixation (retro-chiasmatic lesion) or to the blind spot (optic nerve lesion)?

enter the superior and inferior poles of the disc (Fig. 1-5). A defect of these bundles may cause one of the following

a) Bjerrum, arcuate, or "scimitar" scotoma (Fig. 1-7): This arcuate portion of the field, at 15° from fixation, is known as "Bjerrum's area"

b) Seidel scotoma (Fig. 1-7): A defect in the proximal portion of the NFB, causing a comma-shaped extension of the blind spot

c) Nasal step (of Rönne) (Fig. 1-7): A defect in the distal portion of the arcuate NFB. Since the superior and inferior arcuate bundles do not cross the horizontal raphe of the temporal retina, a nasal step defect respects the horizontal (180°) meridian

d) Isolated scotoma within Bjerrum's area (Fig. 1-7): defect of the intermediate portion of the arcuate NFB

3) Nasal nerve fiber bundles: fibers that enter the nasal aspect of the disc

7

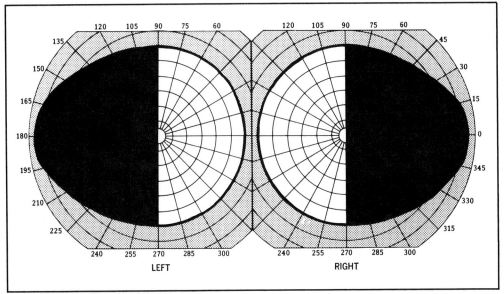

Fig. 1-9. Bitemporal hemianopia due to interruption of decussating nasal fibers in chiasm.

course in a straight (nonarcuate) fashion. The defect in this bundle results in a wedge-shaped temporal scotoma arising from the blind spot and does not necessarily respect the temporal horizontal meridian (Fig. 1-7)

c. Lesions at or behind the chiasm tend to cause hemianopic field defects originating from the fixation point and respecting the vertical meridian

d. Optic nerve lesions cause field defects corresponding to one of the three major NFB defects described above. Nerve fiber bundle defects originate from the blind spot, not from the fixation point, and do not respect the vertical meridian, but do respect the nasal horizontal meridian

e. The KEY QUESTION, therefore, in a patient with a quadrantic field defect is: does the field defect go to fixation or to the blind spot (Fig. 1-8)?

f. Additional clinical findings supporting the diagnosis of optic neuropathy as the cause of the field defect include

    1) Decreased visual acuity: patients with isolated retrochiasmatic lesions do not have decreased visual acuity, unless the lesions are bilateral, and then the visual acuities will be equal; if a patient has hemianopic field defects with unequal visual acuities, then look for a lesion around the chiasm (affecting the optic nerves asymmetrically)

    2) Patients with decreased (or suspected decreased) visual acuity can be further tested with

        a) Light-brightness comparison (eye with optic neuropathy will see the light as "less bright")

        b) Color perception comparison (color plates or Mydriacyl bottle cap) (eye with optic neuropathy will have diminished color perception)

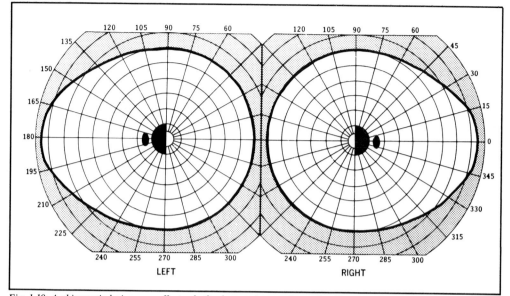

Fig. 1-10. A chiasmatic lesion may affect only the decussating nasal-macular fibers, resulting in a "central bitemporal hemianopia." Therefore, a "complete" visual field evaluation, in a patient suspected of a chiasmatic lesion, must include search of the central field.

    c) Light-stress recovery time (eye with maculopathy will have delayed recovery of visual acuity after bleaching with light)

    d) Afferent pupillary defect test ("Swinging Flashlight" or "Marcus Gunn" test—see Chapter 8)

    e) Tests (a) through (d) may help in distinguishing cases of decreased visual acuity due to macular disease from those due to optic nerve disease

    f) Visually Evoked Potential (VEP)

    g) Ophthalmoscopic evidence of optic disc abnormality e.g. pallor, cupping, drusen

2. "Rules of the Road" for the Optic Chiasm

    a. Three "rules" describe the course of major fiber bundles in the chiasm

        1) The nasal retinal fibers (including the nasal half of the macula) of each eye cross in the chiasm, to the contralateral optic tract. Temporal fibers remain uncrossed. Thus, a chiasmal lesion will cause a bitemporal hemianopia due to interruption of decussating nasal fibers (Fig. 1-9)

        2) Lower retinal fibers project through the optic nerve and chiasm to lie laterally in the tracts; upper retinal fibers will lie medially (there is a 90° rotation of fibers from the nerves through chiasm into the tracts)

        3) Inferonasal retinal fibers cross in the chiasm, and course anteriorly approximately 4mm in the contralateral optic nerve (knee of von Wilbrand) before turning back to join uncrossed inferotemporal fibers in the optic tract (junctional scotoma—see below)

    b. "Macular" crossing fibers are distributed throughout the chiasm, and if

9

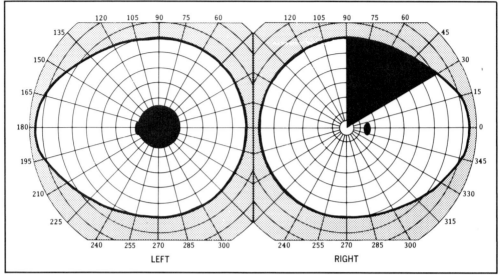

Fig. 1-11. Junctional Scotoma: a central scotoma in one eye with a superior-temporal defect in the fellow eye; indicates a lesion at the "junction" of the optic nerve (L.E., in this case) and the chiasm.

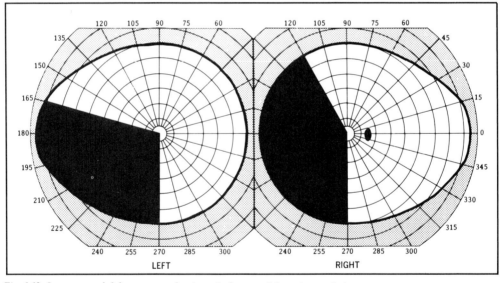

Fig. 1-12. Incongruous left homonymous hemianopia due to a right optic tract lesion.

primarily affected, cause a "central bitemporal hemianopia" (Fig. 1-10)

c. J. Lawton Smith Super Gem: If a patient comes in with poor vision in the LEFT eye, the important eye for visual field exam is the RIGHT. There may be an upper temporal defect with respect for the vertical meridian on the right, due to involvement of von Wilbrand's knee. The lesion is now intracranial at the junction of the left optic nerve and chiasm. The field defects constitute a junctional scotoma (Fig. 1-11)

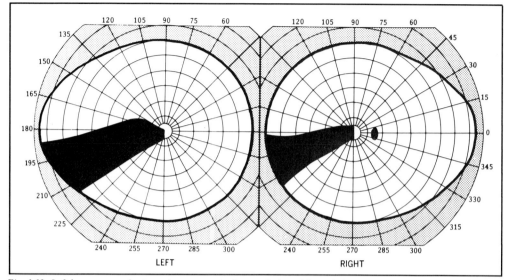

Fig. 1-13. Left homonymous horizontal sectoranopia due to a lesion of the right lateral geniculate nucleus.

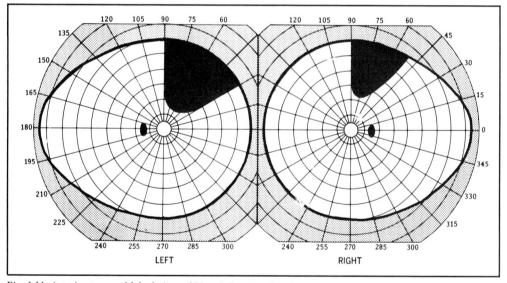

Fig. 1-14. Anterior temporal lobe lesions of Meyer's Loop produce incongruous, mid-peripheral-and-peripheral, contralateral, homonymous, superior ("Pie in the Sky") quadrantanopia. This is an example of a patient with a LEFT temporal lobe lesion.

3. Optic Tract-Lateral Geniculate Body Defects
   a. All retrochiasmatic lesions result in a contralateral homonymous hemianopia
   b. Congruity describes incomplete homonymous hemianopic defects that are identical in all attributes: location, shape, size, depth, slope of margins
   c. REMEMBER: The more posterior (toward the occipital cortex) the lesion in

11

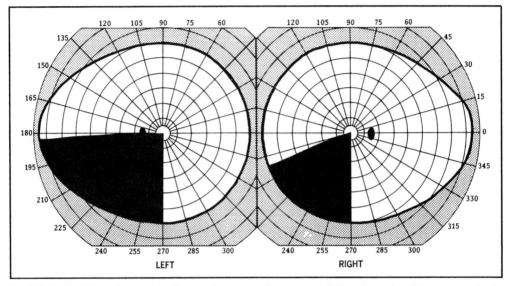

Fig. 1-15. Parietal lobe lesions tend to affect the inferior, contralateral, visual-field quadrants first. This is an example of a patient with a RIGHT parietal lobe lesion.

the post-chiasmal visual pathways, the more likely are the defects to be congruous

d. In the optic tracts and lateral geniculate body, nerve fibers of corresponding points (retinal positions of the two eyes that image the same position in visual space) do not yet lie adjacent to one another. This leads to incongruous visual field defects (Fig. 1-12)

e. Criteria for optic tract syndrome
   1) Incongruous homonymous hemianopia
   2) Bilateral retinal nerve fiber layer atrophy or optic (occasionally "bowtie") atrophy
   3) Pupillary abnormalities
      a) relative afferent defect: on side opposite the lesion (eye with temporal field loss)
      b) Wernicke's pupil: light stimulation of "blind" retina causes no pupillary reaction, while light projected on "intact" retina produces normal pupillary constriction
      c) Behr's pupil: anisocoria with larger pupil on side of hemianopia; probably does not exist

f. Lateral geniculate body field defect
   1) Extremely rare
   2) Two types of defects
      a) incongruous homonymous hemianopia
      b) relatively congruous homonymous horizontal sectoranopia (Fig. 1-13): associated with sectorial optic atrophy; may be due to vascular infarction of a portion of the lateral geniculate body

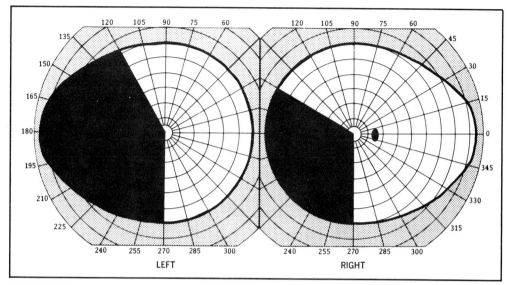

Fig. 1-16. INCONGRUOUS Left Homonymous Hemianopia.

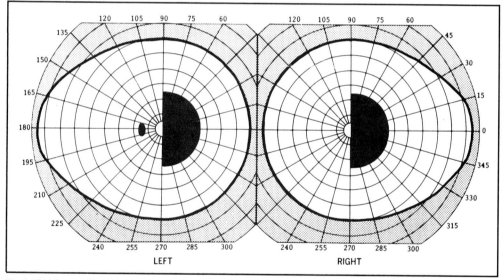

Fig. 1-17. A lesion affecting only the tip of the occipital lobe produces a defect of only the central homonymous hemi-fields. This is an example of a patient with a LEFT occipital-tip lesion.

4. Superior-Inferior Separation in the Temporal Lobe
   a. Inferior fibers (ipsilateral inferotemporal fibers and contralateral inferonasal fibers) course anteriorly from the lateral geniculate body into the temporal lobe, forming Meyer's loop, approximately 2.5 cm from the anterior tip of the temporal lobe. They are anatomically separated from the superior retinal fibers which course directly back in the optic radiations of the parietal lobe (Fig. 1-4)

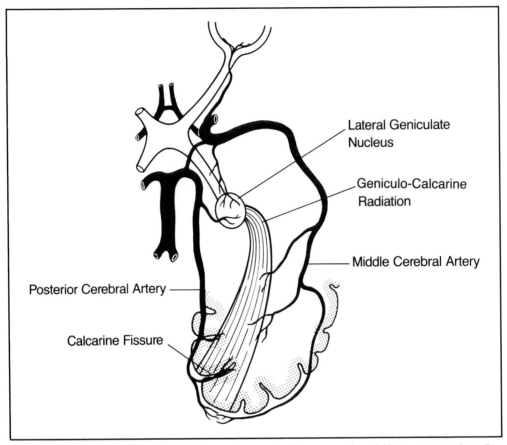

Fig. 1-18. The tip of the occipital lobe, where the macular or central homonymous hemi-fields are represented (see Fig. 1-4), is supplied by TERMINAL branches of the MIDDLE AND POSTERIOR Cerebral Arteries; it is referred to as a WATERSHED area. The mesial surface of the occipital lobe is supplied by more proximal (NOT TERMINAL) branches of the POSTERIOR Cerebral Artery.

    b. Inferior "macular" fibers do not cross as far anteriorly in the temporal lobe

    c. Anterior temporal lobe lesions tend to produce mid-peripheral and peripheral contralateral homonymous superior quadrantanopia ("pie in the sky" field defect) (Fig. 1-14)

    d. More extensive temporal lobe lesions may cause field defects that extend to the inferior quadrants, but hemianopia will be "denser" superiorly

5. Superior-Inferior Separation in the Parietal Lobe

    a. Superior fibers (ipsilateral superotemporal fibers and contralateral superonasal fibers) cross directly through the parietal lobe to lie superiorly in the optic radiation

    b. Inferior fibers course through the temporal lobe (Meyer's Loop) and lie inferiorly in the optic radiation

    c. Thus, there is "correction" of the 90° rotation of the visual fibers that occurred through the chiasm into the tracts

    d. Parietal lobe lesions tend to affect superior fibers first, resulting in con-

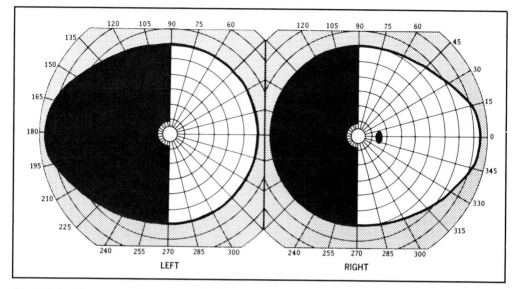

Fig. 1-19. Left Homonymous Hemianopia with "SPARING" of the left half of the macular field of each eye.

tralateral inferior homonymous quadrantanopia (Fig. 1-15) or a homonymous hemianopia "denser" inferiorly (Fig. 1-16)
   e. Two signs described with parietal lobe lesions
      1) Spasticity of conjugate gaze: tonic deviation of eyes to side opposite a parietal lesion during an attempt to produce Bell's phenomenon (see Chapter 2)
      2) Optokinetic nystagmus asymmetry: evoked nystagmus is dampened when stimuli are moved in the direction of the damaged parietal lobe (see below—"rule" 9)
6. Central Homonymous Hemianopia
   a. In the visual cortex, the macular representation is located on the tips of the occipital lobes
   b. The macular representation is separated from the cortical representation of the midperipheral and peripheral visual fields. These fibers terminate on the mesial surface of the occipital lobes (Fig. 1-4)
   c. A lesion affecting the tip of the occipital lobe tends to produce a central homonymous hemianopia (Fig. 1-17)
7. Macular Sparing
   a. The macular area of the visual cortex is a watershed area with respect to blood supply (Fig. 1-18)
      1) The "macular" visual cortex is supplied by terminal branches of posterior and middle cerebral arteries
      2) The visual cortex subserving midperipheral and peripheral field is supplied only by the posterior cerebral artery. The area is supplied by a more proximal (not a terminal) vessel
      3) Therefore, when there is obstruction of flow through the posterior

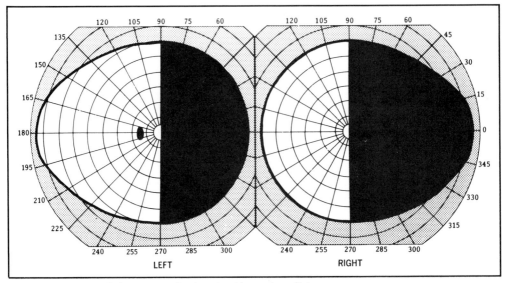

Fig. 1-20. Complete right homonymous hemianopia with macular splitting.

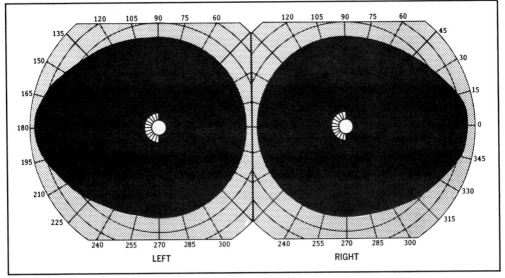

Fig. 1-21. Bilateral homonymous hemianopias with macular sparing.

cerebral artery, ipsilateral macular visual cortex may be spared, because of blood supply provided by the terminal branches of the middle cerebral artery. This may be an explanation for "macular sparing"

4) However, when there is a generalized hypoperfusion state (e.g. intra-operative hypotension) the first area of the visual cortex to be affected is that supplied by terminal branches, the macular visual cortex, resulting in a central homonymous hemianopia (see Fig. 1-17)

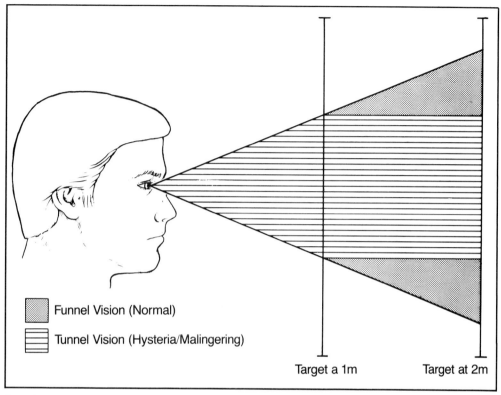

Funnel Vision (Normal)

Tunnel Vision (Hysteria/Malingering)

Target a 1m   Target at 2m

Fig. 1-22

b. In order to qualify as "macular sparing," at least 5° of the macular field must be spared in both eyes, on the side of the hemianopia (Fig. 1-19)

c. Macular sparing may actually be an artifact of testing. The patient may shift fixation, anticipating the appearance of the test object

d. If a patient with a complete homonymous hemianopia is found to have sparing of the macula, then he is most likely to have an occipital lobe lesion; however, a majority of patients with occipital lobe lesions demonstrate a splitting of the macula (Fig. 1-20); therefore, "macular sparing" is helpful only if present

e. Bilateral homonymous hemianopias with macular sparing produce constricted visual fields (with normal fundi) (Fig. 1-21). The differential diagnosis of constricted visual fields also includes:
   1) hysteria/malingering
   2) glaucoma
   3) optic disc drusen
   4) post-papilledema optic atrophy
   5) retinitis pigmentosa

f. Items two through five listed above all have abnormal fundi and should be easily diagnosed. Differential from hysteria/malingering requires visual fields done at the tangent screen at 1 and 2 meters (Fig. 1-22)

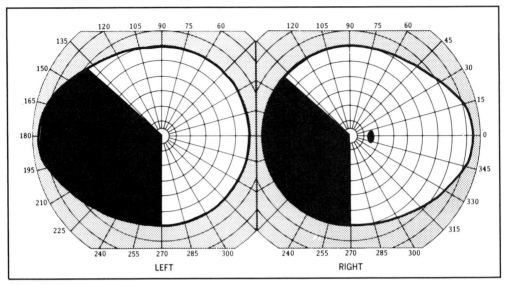

Fig. 1-23. Congruous left homonymous hemianopia.

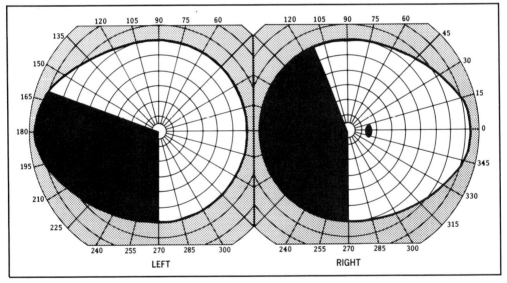

Fig. 1-24. Incongruous left homonymous hemianopia.

8. Congruity
   a. Homonymous hemianopic field defects are said to be congruous when the defect is not complete (i.e. does not occupy the entire half of the field) and the defect extends to the same angular meridian in both eyes (Fig. 1-23; the hemianopia defect extends to the 137° meridian in each eye)
   b. Complete homonymous hemianopia (Fig. 1-20) cannot be categorized by "congruity," because it is complete
   c. Figure 1-24 shows an example of incongruity, the hemianopia of the left eye

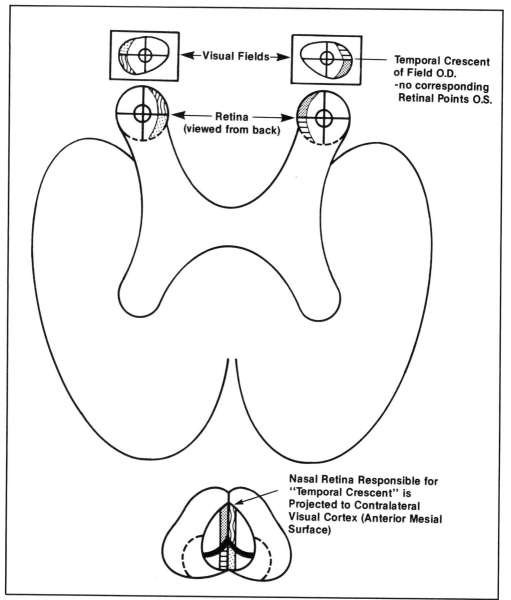

Fig. 1-25. Temporal crescent.

extending to the 160° meridian while the hemianopia of the right eye extends to the 115° meridian

    d. Optic tract lesions tend to produce markedly incongruous field defects

    e. The more congruous a homonymous hemianopia is, the nearer the lesion will be to the occipital cortex (i.e., more posterior in the visual pathways)

    f. Congruity is due to the fact that a lesion affects nerve fibers from corresponding retinal points which lie adjacent to one another

9. Optokinetic Nystagmus (OKN)

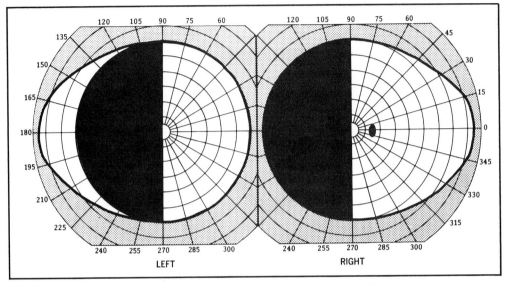

Fig. 1-26. Left Homonymous Hemianopia with sparing of the temporal crescent of the left eye.

a. The precise pathways of the optokinetic system are unknown in humans, but may share pathways carrying smooth pursuit commands. This pathway extends from the visual association areas (18 and 19) to the horizontal gaze center in the pons (see Chapter 2)

b. The pathway in the left visual association area will terminate in the left pontine gaze center, resulting in pursuit movement of the eyes to the left. Similarly, the pathway originating in the right cerebral hemisphere generates pursuit eye movements to the right

c. A patient with a purely occipital lobe lesion (even if resulting in a complete homonymous hemianopia) will have no difficulty with pursuit, since the pathways begin more anteriorly. OKN response will be symmetric (see Fig. 2-8)

d. A patient with homonymous hemianopia due to a parietal lobe lesion will have deficient pursuit eye movements to the side of the lesion, resulting in asymmetric OKN. The OKN will be decreased when the drum is rotated toward the side of the lesion (see Fig. 2-9)

e. Patients with homonymous hemianopia due to an optic tract, temporal lobe, or purely occipital lobe lesion will have symmetric OKN to both sides

f. Cogan's Dictum

1) Homonymous hemianopia + asymmetric OKN . . . probably parietal lobe lesion . . . most likely mass

2) Homonymous hemianopia + symmetric OKN . . . probably occipital lobe lesion . . . most likely vascular infarction

10. Temporal Crescent

a. When we fixate with both eyes and achieve fusion of the visual information gained by both eyes, there is superimposition of the corresponding portions of the visual fields: the central 50° radius of field in each eye

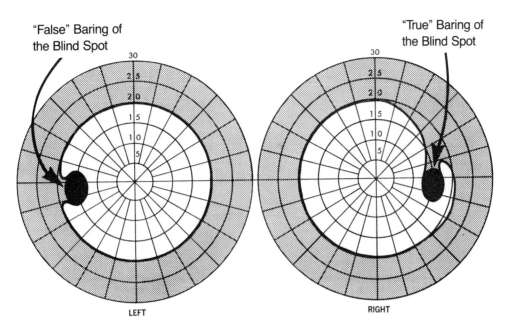

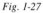

Fig. 1-27

b. There remains, in each eye, a temporal crescent of field for which there are no corresponding visual points in the other eye (Fig. 1-25)

c. This temporal crescent of field, perceived by a nasal crescent of retina, is represented in the contralateral visual cortex, in the most anterior portion of the mesial surface of the occipital lobe (along the calcarine fissure)

d. If a patient is found to have a homonymous hemianopia with sparing of the temporal crescent (Fig. 1-26), then he probably has an occipital lobe lesion, since this is the only site where the temporal crescent of fibers are separated from the other nasal fibers of the contralateral eye

H. Special Visual Field Cases

1. Baring of the Blind Spot
   a. "Baring" of the blind spot in glaucoma: when a small isopter is being studied (e.g. 25° radius, the field thus being just outside the blind spot, which is 15-20° from fixation) the patient with Seidel scotoma (Fig. 1-7) may demonstrate a connection between the blind spot and non-seeing area outside 25° radius (Fig. 1-27); this is "true" baring of the blind spots
   b. A normal patient may exhibit "false" baring of the blind spot when the isopter is "just" outside the blind spot (Fig. 1-27)

2. Pseudo-bitemporal Hemianopia
   a. Field defects that do not respect vertical meridian, but rather "slope" across it (Fig. 1-28)
   b. Causes include
      1) uncorrected refractive errors (myopia, astigmatism)
      2) titled optic discs

21

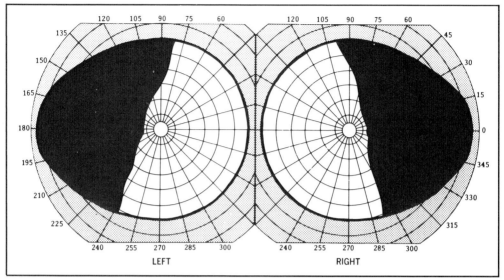

Fig. 1-28. Pseudo-bitemporal hemianopia. Field defects do not respect the vertical meridian.

    3) enlarged blind spots in papilledema
    4) large central or centrocecal scotomas
    5) sectoral retinitis pigmentosa (mainly in nasal quadrants)
    6) overhanging eyelid tissue
3. Binasal Hemianopia
  a. Most nasal field defects are due to arcuate scotomas
  b. Rarely, true unilateral or bilateral nasal hemianopia may occur with defects having no arcuate connection to the blind spot and, to some extent, respecting the vertical meridian
  c. Never as a result of chiasmal compression
  d. May be due to pressure upon the temporal aspect of the optic nerve and the anterior angle of the chiasm or near the optic canal; in these locations a lesion may affect only temporal retinal fibers. The fibers cannot be selectively obstructed in the lateral chiasm
  e. Cause includes aneurysm, tumor (pituitary adenoma), vascular infarction

Bibliography

BOOKS
Anderson DR: Testing the Field of Vision. St. Louis, CV Mosby, 1982.
Harrington DO: The Visual Fields, ed 4. St. Louis, CV Mosby, 1976.
Traquair HM: Clinical Perimetry, ed 7. London, Henry Kimpton, 1957.
Trobe JD, Glaser JS: The Visual Fields Manual. Gainesville, Triad Publishing Co., 1982.

CHAPTERS
Glaser JS: Neuro-ophthalmology, in Duane TD (ed). Clinical Ophthalmology, Hagerstown, Harper & Row, 1978, Vol. 2, Chapters 4-7, pp. 49-167.
Hollenhorst RW, Younge BR: Ocular manifestations produced by adenomas of the pituitary gland: Analysis

of 1000 cases, in Kohler DO, Ross GT (eds): Diagnosis and treatment of pituitary tumors. Amsterdam, Excerpta Medica, 1973, pp. 53-64.

Miller NR: Walsh and Hoyt's Clinical Neuro-ophthalmology. Baltimore, Williams & Wilkins, 1982, Chapters 1-11, pp. 3-171.

ARTICLES

Frisén L: Quadruple sectoranopia and sectorial optic atrophy: a syndrome of the distal anterior choroidal artery. J Neurol Neurosurg Psychiatry 1979; 42:590-594.

Frisén L, Holmegaard L, Rosencrantz M: Sectorial optic atrophy and homonymous, horizontal sectoranopia: a lateral choroidal artery syndrome? J Neurol Neurosurg Psychiatry 1978; 41:374-380.

Hoyt WF, Luis O: The primate chiasm: Details of visual fiber organization studied by silver impregnation techniques. Arch Ophthalmol 1962; 68:94-106.

Hoyt WF, Tudor RC: The course of parapapillary temporal retinal axons through the anterior optic nerve. A Nanta degeneration study in the primate. Arch Ophthalmol 1963; 69:503-507.

Salinas RF, Smith JL: Binasal hemianopia. Surg Neurol 1978; 10:187-194.

Savino PJ, Paris M, Schatz NJ et al: Optic tract syndrome. Arch Ophthalmol 1978; 96:656-663.

Smith JL: Homonymous hemianopia: a review of one hundred cases. Am J Ophthalmol 1962; 54:616-623.

Smith JL, Cogan DG: Optokinetic nystagmus: a test for parietal lobe lesions. Am J Ophthalmol 1959; 48:187-193.

Trobe JD, Lorber ML, Schlezinger NS: Isolated homonymous hemianopsias: a review of 104 cases. Arch Ophthalmol 1973; 89:377-381.

Van Buren JM, Baldwin M: The architecture of the optic radiation in the temporal lobe of man. Brain 1958; 81:15-40.

Visual Field Quiz

1. Test yourself in the interpretation of the following hypothetical cases (Figures E1-E33).
2. Unless stated otherwise, assume that the visual fields have been evaluated with a perimeter, using the same stimulus and testing conditions for each eye.

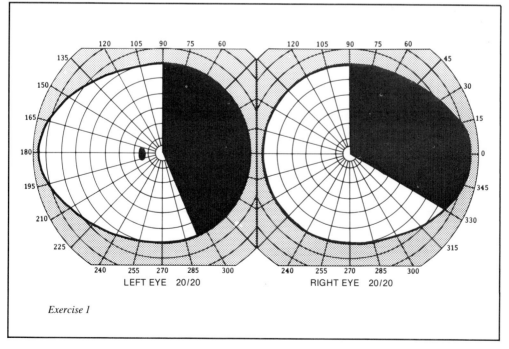

LEFT EYE 20/20   RIGHT EYE 20/20

Exercise 1

3. Describe and categorize the visual field defects and suggest the probable localization and possible causes of the lesion(s).
4. Develop a systematic approach that includes a review of the "Ten Key Points to Remember."
5. Remember the significance of altered visual acuities (see Section G, 1, f).

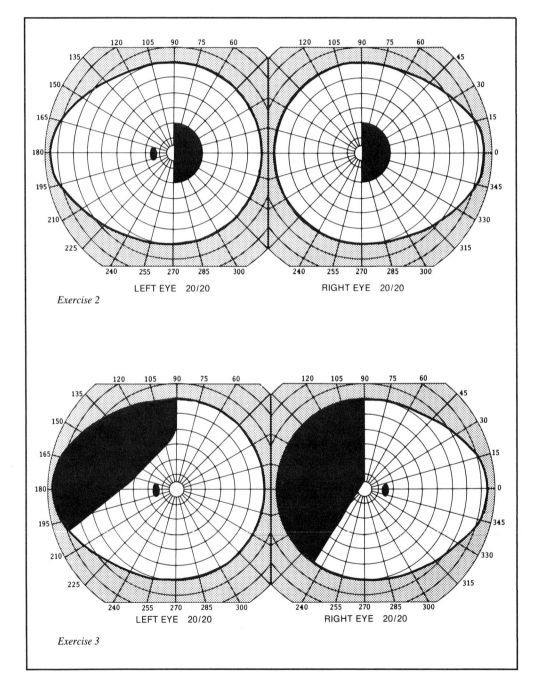

Exercise 2

LEFT EYE   20/20   RIGHT EYE   20/20

Exercise 3

LEFT EYE   20/20   RIGHT EYE   20/20

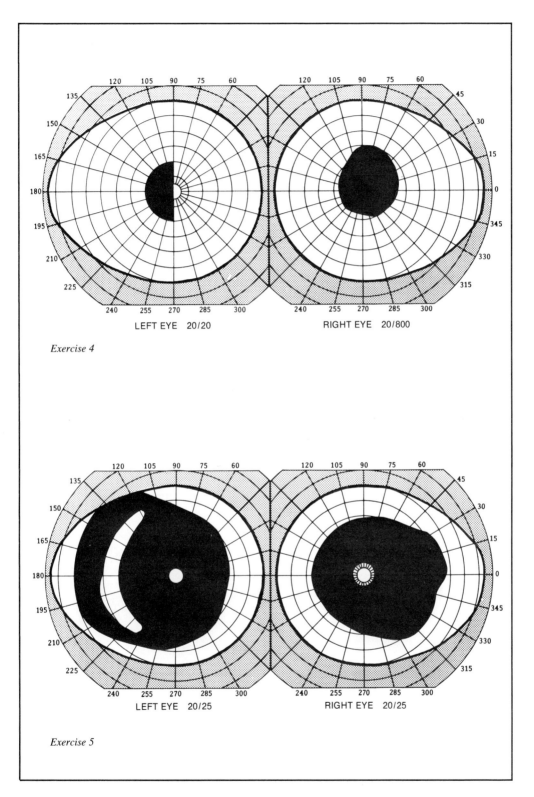

LEFT EYE   20/20   RIGHT EYE   20/800

Exercise 4

LEFT EYE   20/25   RIGHT EYE   20/25

Exercise 5

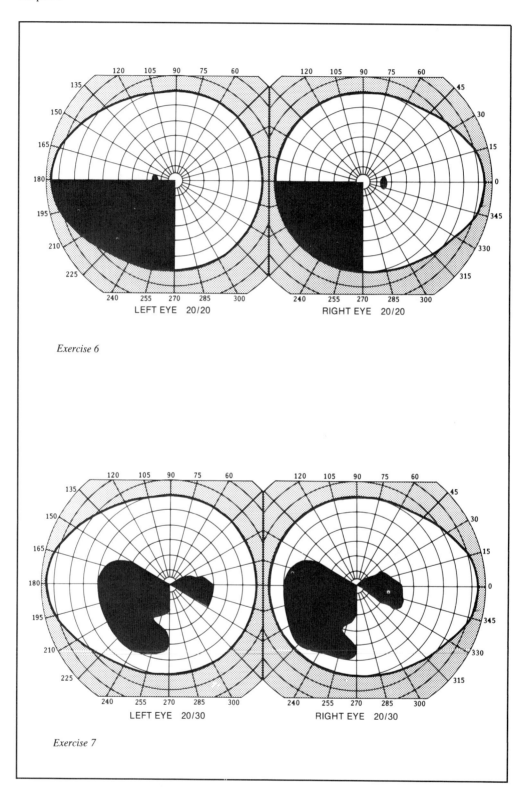

Exercise 6

Exercise 7

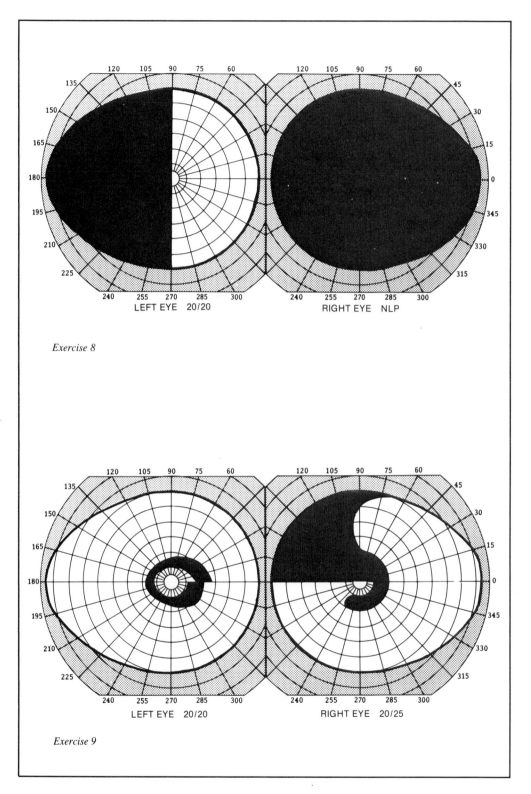

LEFT EYE   20/20

RIGHT EYE   NLP

Exercise 8

LEFT EYE   20/20

RIGHT EYE   20/25

Exercise 9

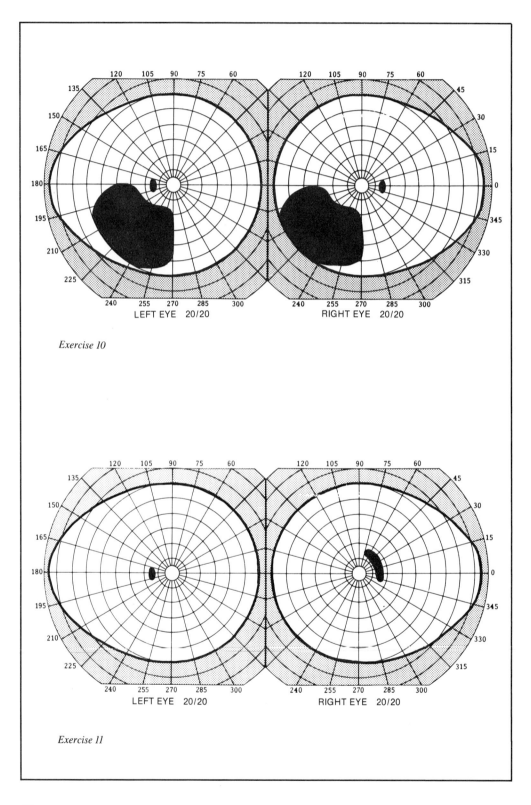

Exercise 10

Exercise 11

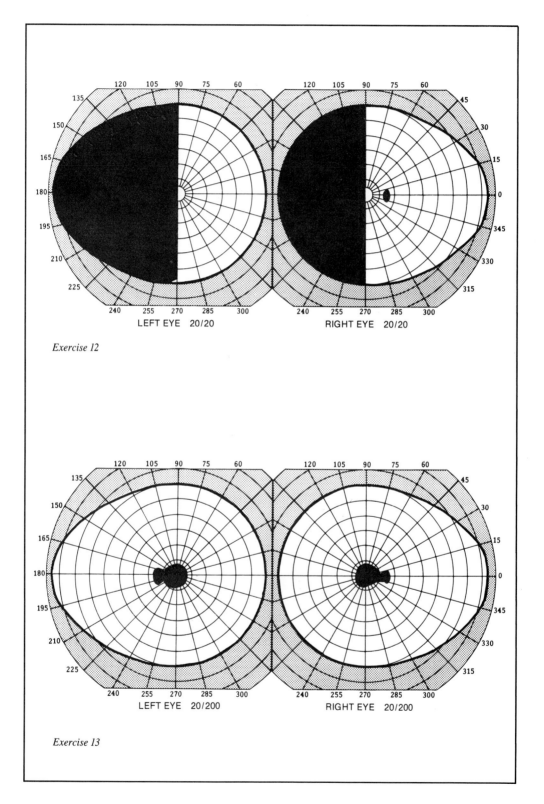

Exercise 12

LEFT EYE   20/20

RIGHT EYE   20/20

Exercise 13

LEFT EYE   20/200

RIGHT EYE   20/200

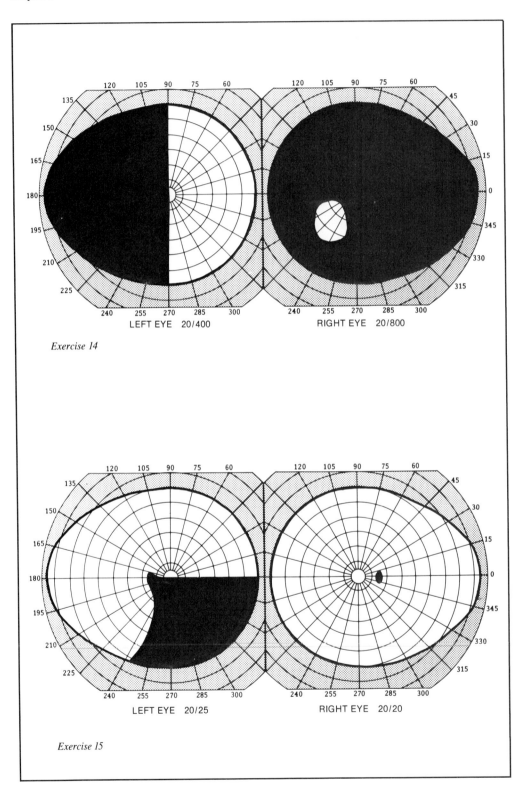

Exercise 14

Exercise 15

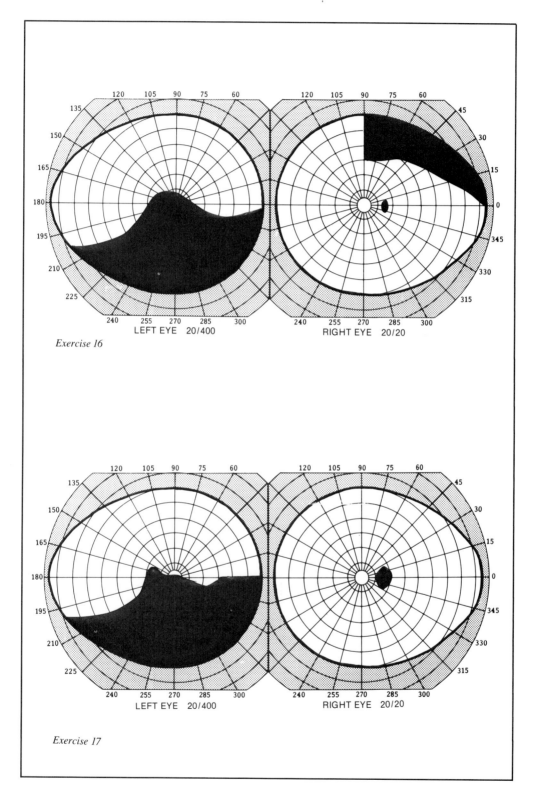

Exercise 16

LEFT EYE   20/400

RIGHT EYE   20/20

Exercise 17

LEFT EYE   20/400

RIGHT EYE   20/20

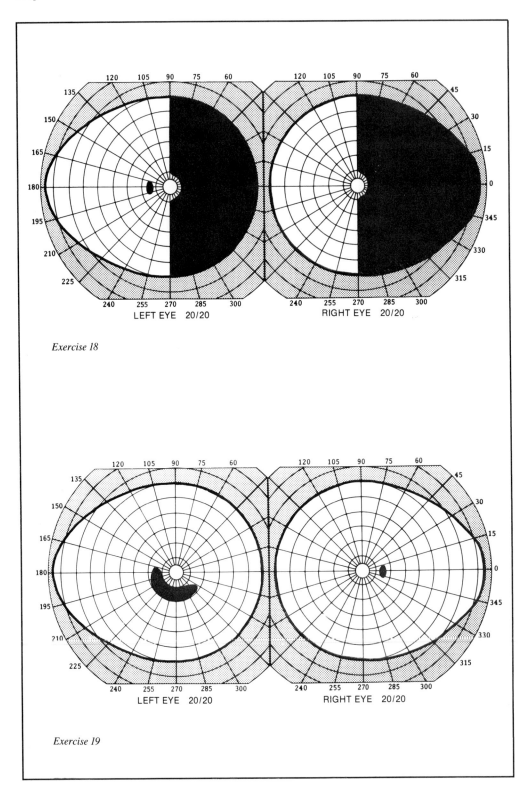

Exercise 18

LEFT EYE 20/20

RIGHT EYE 20/20

Exercise 19

LEFT EYE 20/20

RIGHT EYE 20/20

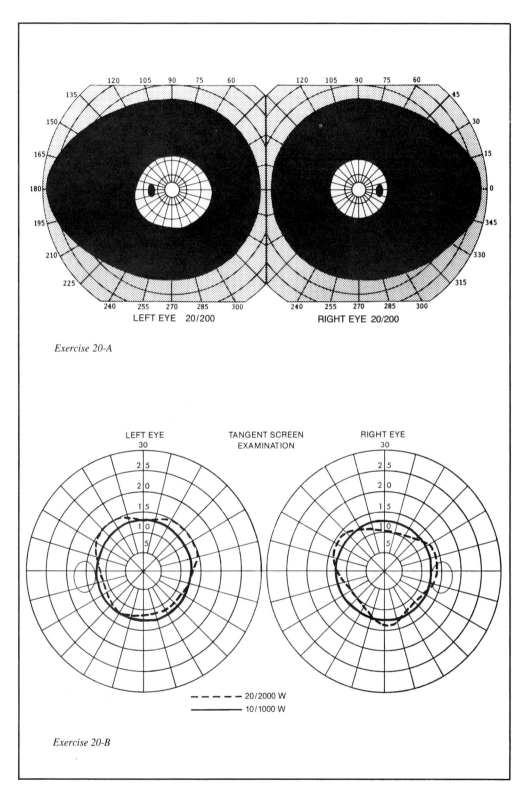

LEFT EYE   20/200

RIGHT EYE   20/200

Exercise 20-A

LEFT EYE
30

TANGENT SCREEN
EXAMINATION

RIGHT EYE
30

- - - - - 20/2000 W
————— 10/1000 W

Exercise 20-B

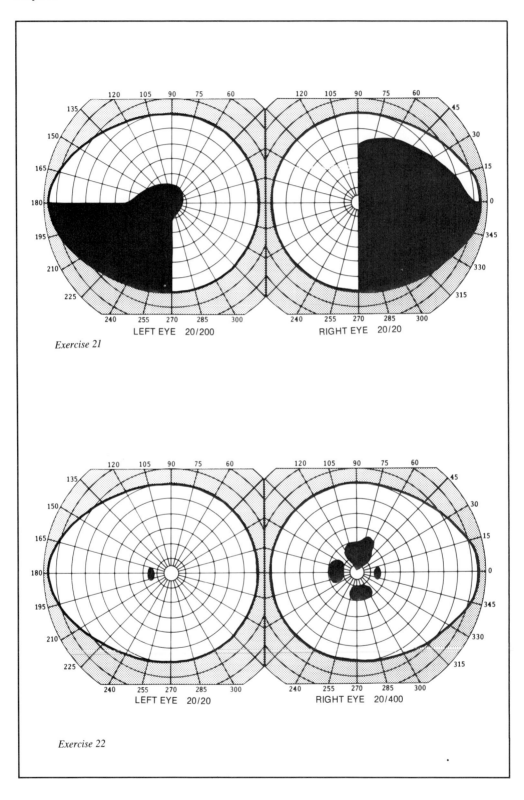

LEFT EYE 20/200

RIGHT EYE 20/20

Exercise 21

LEFT EYE 20/20

RIGHT EYE 20/400

Exercise 22

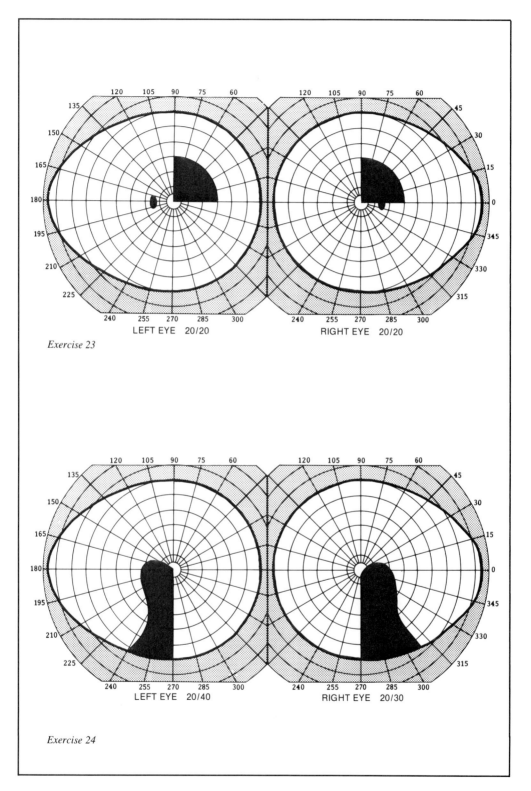

Exercise 23

LEFT EYE   20/20

RIGHT EYE   20/20

Exercise 24

LEFT EYE   20/40

RIGHT EYE   20/30

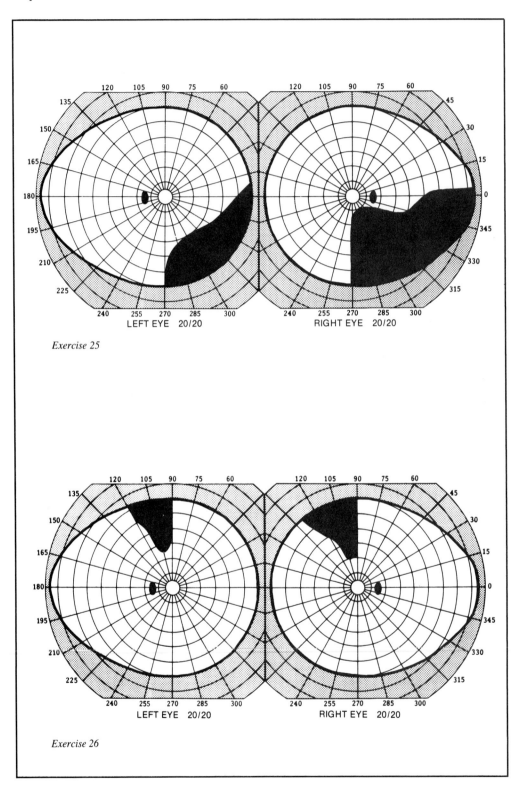

LEFT EYE 20/20   RIGHT EYE 20/20

Exercise 25

LEFT EYE 20/20   RIGHT EYE 20/20

Exercise 26

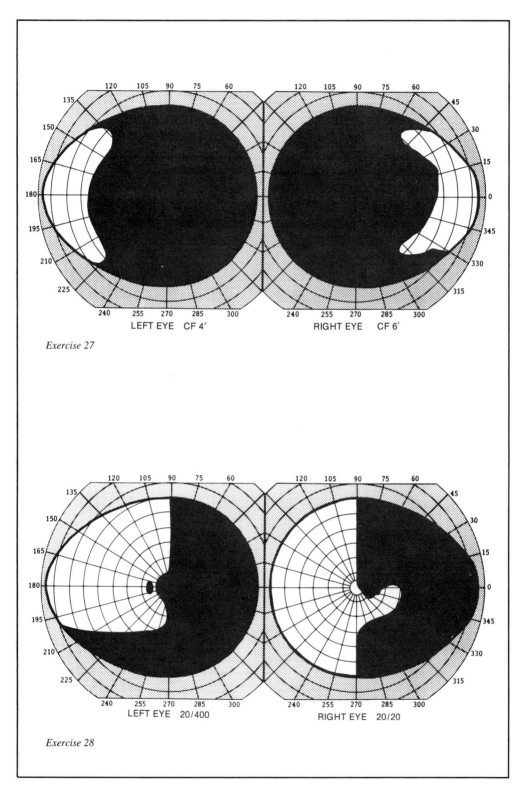

Exercise 27

LEFT EYE   CF 4′

RIGHT EYE   CF 6′

Exercise 28

LEFT EYE   20/400

RIGHT EYE   20/20

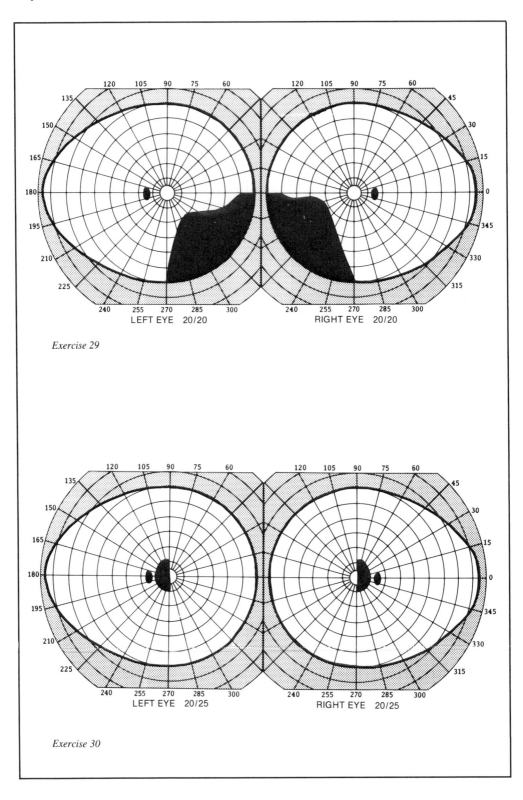

Exercise 29

Exercise 30

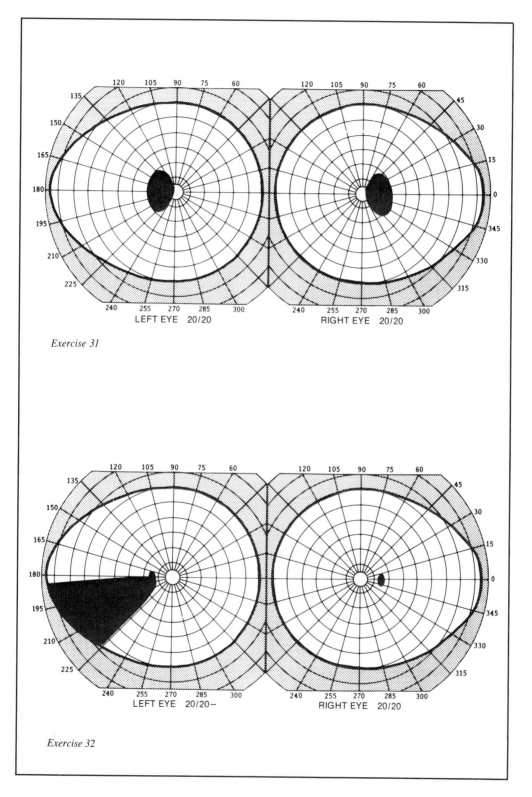

Exercise 31

LEFT EYE 20/20

RIGHT EYE 20/20

Exercise 32

LEFT EYE 20/20−

RIGHT EYE 20/20

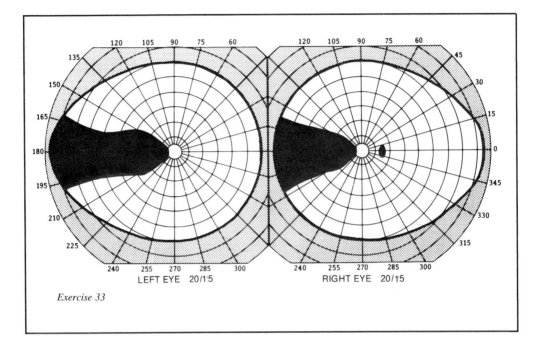

LEFT EYE 20/15   RIGHT EYE 20/15

Exercise 33

Plausible Interpretations of the Mystery Visual Field Defects

E1. R Homonymous Hemianopia, incongruous, denser above, but extending to fixation and into the inferior quadrants.
L temporal lobe lesion extending to the L parietal lobe.

E2. R Homonymous Hemianopia, central (macular), congruous.
L occipital tip.

E3. L Homonymous Hemianopia, denser above, markedly incongruous. Marked incongruity suggests possibility of R optic tract lesion, but greater density above suggests possibility of R temporal lobe lesion, which would also be 10 times more likely, statistically.

E4. R central scotoma; L central (macular) temporal hemianopia.
R optic nerve lesion at the junction of the nerve to the chiasm.

E5. Bilateral ring scotomas, with preservation of central 10 to 20 degrees with vision of 20/25, OU.
Retinitis pigmentosa versus advanced glaucoma.

E6. L Homonymous Inferior Quadrantanopia, congruous.
R Parietal versus Occipital lesion. The congruity gives the edge to the occipital localization.

E7. Bilateral, incomplete homonymous hemianopias, congruous.
Bilateral occipital lesions.

E8. Blind OD with temporal hemianopia OS.
R optic nerve lesion extending into the chiasm.

E9. Double Bjerrum scotoma OS, creating a "ring" scotoma. OD: Inferior arcuate scotoma (incomplete Bjerrum scotoma); superior Bjerrum scotoma breaking

through nasally to create a peripheral nasal step of Rönne.
Glaucoma.

E10. L Homonymous inferior quadrantanopia, congruous, with sparing of temporal crescent, OS, and bilateral macular sparing.
R Occipital lesion, upper bank of the calcarine fissure.

E11. R superior Seidel scotoma.
Glaucoma. Expect to see inferior elongation of the right cup.

E12. L Homonymous Hemianopia, complete (cannot make statement about congruity).
R optic tract, parietal, or occipital lesion. OKN asymmetry would identify the parietal cases.

E13. Bilateral centrocecal scotomas.
Bilateral optic neuropathy.

E14. Inferior nasal island remaining OD. Temporal hemianopia with involvement of central field OS.
Extensive chiasmatic lesion.

E15. Inferior ("fat" Bjerrum scotoma) altitudinal defect OS. OD normal.
OS optic nerve lesion: glaucoma versus Ischemic Optic Neuropathy (ION).

E16. Inferior ("fat" Bjerrum scotoma) altitudinal defect OS, with involvement of central field. Superior temporal cut OD.
Lesion at junction of L optic nerve and chiasm (Junctional Scotoma).

E17. Inferior ("fat" Bjerrum scotoma) altitudinal defect OS, with involvement of the central field. Enlarged blind spot OD. Intracranial left optic nerve lesion. We suspect that the lesion is intracranial because the right optic disc appears to be edematous, probably due to increased intracranial pressure caused by the left optic nerve tumor (meningioma?). Expect to see the disc changes associated with the Foster Kennedy syndrome (optic atrophy OS and disc edema OD).

E18. R Homonymous Hemianopia, complete, with macular sparing.
L occipital cortex.

E19. Inferior arcuate scotoma (Nerve Fiber Bundle Defect; incomplete Bjerrum scotoma) OS. OD normal.
Look for disc changes. Superior elongation of the cup (glaucoma). Lumpy disc (drusen).

E20. Tubular fields, with discrepancy of size of remaining fields when comparing perimeter (20-A) and tangent screen (20-B) fields. "Tunnel" vision.
Psychogenic field defects.

E21. Bitemporal hemianopia with central scotoma OS.
Chiasm.

E22. Multiple central and paracentral defects OD. OS normal.
Retinal lesions (chorioretinitis).

E23. R Homonymous superior quadrantanopia, congruous, central, involving macular field.
L occipital tip, inferior calcarine cortex.

E24. Bitemporal inferior quadrantanopia.
Chiasmatic lesion with some involvement of the crossed macular fibers, causing slightly decreased acuities.

E25. R Homonymous, inferior quadrantanopia, markedly incongruous.
L parietal versus L optic tract.

E26. L homonymous superior quadrantanopia, incongruous. "Pie in the Sky" defects.
R temporal lobe (Meyer's Loop) lesion.

E27. Temporal islands remaining OU.
End-stage Glaucoma.

E28. R Homonymous Hemianopia, incongruous, with central scotoma OS.
L optic tract lesion at junction of tract and chiasm, affecting some of the crossing macular fibers of the left eye, causing decreased acuity in that eye.

E29. Bilateral inferior nasal contraction.
Optic nerve or retinal lesions (optic disc drusen, glaucoma, retinoschisis).

E30. Bitemporal Hemianopia, central (macular).
Chiasm.

E31. Enlarged blind spots OU, causing Pseudo-Bitemporal Hemianopia.
Papilledema.

E32. Inferior-temporal wedge-shaped field defect OS. OD normal. A Nerve Fiber Bundle Defect affecting the superior-nasal bundle of nerve fibers (see Figs. 1-5, 1-7).
An uncommon, but well-documented, glaucomatous field defect. May represent the residual of papillitis.

E33. Congruous horizontal wedge-shaped left sectoranopia, a rare field defect due to a lesion of right lateral geniculate nucleus.

2

Supranuclear and Internuclear Gaze Pathways

A. The eyes move in six ways, two of them fast and four of them slow
  1. Fast Eye Movements (FEM) (velocity: 300-700°/second)
     a. saccade (French term for "jerk movement")
     b. nystagmus quick phase
  2. Slow Eye Movements (SEM) (velocity: 20-50°/second)
     a. smooth pursuit
     b. optokinetic
     c. vestibular
     d. vergence
B. Functional Classification of Eye Movements

TABLE 2-1
A FUNCTIONAL CLASSIFICATION OF HUMAN EYE MOVEMENTS*

Class of Eye Movements	Main Function
Saccades	To bring images of objects of interest onto the fovea
Nystagmus quick phases	To direct the fovea toward the oncoming visual scene during self-rotation; to reset the eyes during prolonged rotation
Smooth pursuit	To hold the image of a moving target on the fovea
Optokinetic	To hold images of the seen world steady on the retina during sustained head rotation
Vestibular (vestibulo-ocular reflex)	To hold images of the seen world steady on the retina during brief head rotations
Vergence	To move the eyes in opposite directions so that images of a single object are placed on both foveae

---

* *Modified from Leigh RJ, Zee DS: The Neurology of Eye Movement. Philadelphia, F.A. Davis Co., 1983, p. 2.*

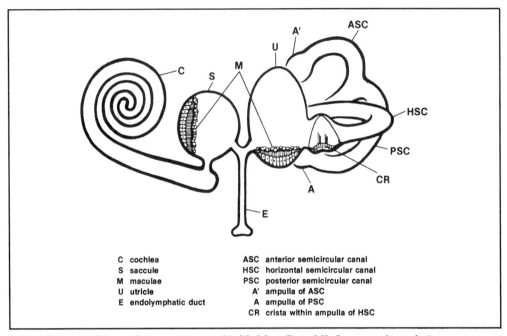

C   cochlea
S   saccule
M   maculae
U   utricle
E   endolymphatic duct

ASC anterior semicircular canal
HSC horizontal semicircular canal
PSC posterior semicircular canal
A' ampulla of ASC
A   ampulla of PSC
CR crista within ampulla of HSC

Fig. 2-1. Diagram of the membranous inner ear. (Modified from Frenzel H: Spontan-und provokations—nystagmus. Basel, S. Krager AG, 1982).

1. FEM: saccades
   a. Stimuli
      1) Voluntary changes in direction
      2) Sudden peripheral-visual, auditory or peripheral-sensory (e.g. pain) stimulus
   b. Saccadic "suppression": even though the visual world is rapidly sweeping across the retina, there is no sense of a blurred image
2. FEM: nystagmus quick phase
   a. Stimulus: sustained head rotation would lead the eyes to extreme contraversive deviation unless prevented by corrective quick phases
   b. This type of FEM is the phylogenetic forerunner of voluntary saccades
3. SEM: smooth pursuit
   a. Stimuli
      1) Motion of the image of a target across the foveal and perifoveal retina
      2) Occasionally the perception of image motion may be insufficient and nonvisual stimuli such as proprioception can also generate smooth pursuit movements
      3) After the eyes have achieved voluntary or involuntary macular fixation of a slowly, smoothly moving target, the eyes will pursue at the velocity of target in a smooth fashion
      4) If the target is moving at a velocity greater than 50°/second, then the eyes, after falling behind in their pursuit, will execute saccadic, voluntary FEM in order to regain macular fixation; the eyes will then pursue

with the smooth SEM until they fall behind again; this results in another "catch-up" saccadic FEM and in the phenomenon of cogwheel pursuit eye movements

4. SEM: optokinetic system
   a. Stimulus: sustained head rotation
   b. Since the vestibular system responds only to acceleration with sustained head rotation (> 30 seconds), this response fades and the optokinetic system maintains compensatory slow-phase eye movements
5. SEM: vestibular
   a. The membranous labyrinth lies within its bony compartment in the temporal bone, cushioned by perilymph (Fig. 2-1)
   b. It contains:
      1) Three semicircular canals and their respective cristae (each in an ampulla) which sense head rotation
      2) The utricle and saccule and their respective maculae which sense head position
   c. The semicircular canals, utricle and saccule contain endolymph
   d. The cristae and maculae contain specialized hair cells that transduce mechanical shearing forces into neural impulses
   e. The vestibular motion sensors detect transient head rotation
   f. Stimulation of each set of semicircular canals precisely influences a particular pair of eye muscles:
      horizontal canals—lateral nystagmus
      posterior canals—vertical nystagmus
      anterior canals—rotary nystagmus
   g. The horizontal semicircular canals are oriented 30° above the horizon, with the ampullae anteriorly located (Fig. 2-2)
   h. In order to maximally affect the horizontal semicircular canals, a specific head position is required (Fig. 2-3)
      1) Head is inclined forward 30° for maximal effect of rotational forces in Barany chair
      2) Head is inclined backward 60° for maximal effect for the convection currents of endolymph flow with caloric testing (Fig. 2-4)
   i. During doll's eye testing, when the head is rotated toward the left side, the endolymph moves toward the left ampulla and away from the right ampulla (Fig. 2-5)
   j. Converse movements of the endolymph occur when the head is rotated to the right side
   k. Movement of the endolymph (by calorics, Barany chair rotation, or doll's eye testing) toward the ampulla result in stimulation of that ampulla
   l. Movement of the endolymph away from the ampulla results in inhibition (lack of stimulation) of that ampulla
6. SEM: vergence
   a. Vergence eye movements are disconjugate; they carry the eyes in opposite directions to direct both foveas at one object of interest

45

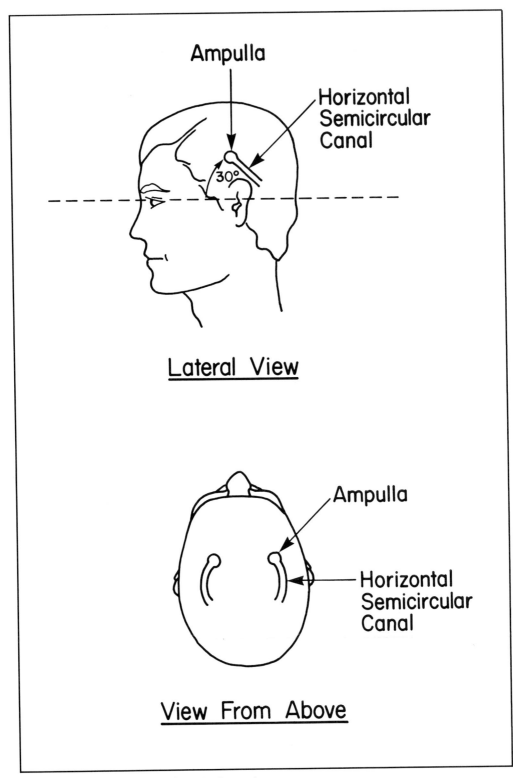

Fig. 2-2. Orientation of the horizontal semicircular canals.

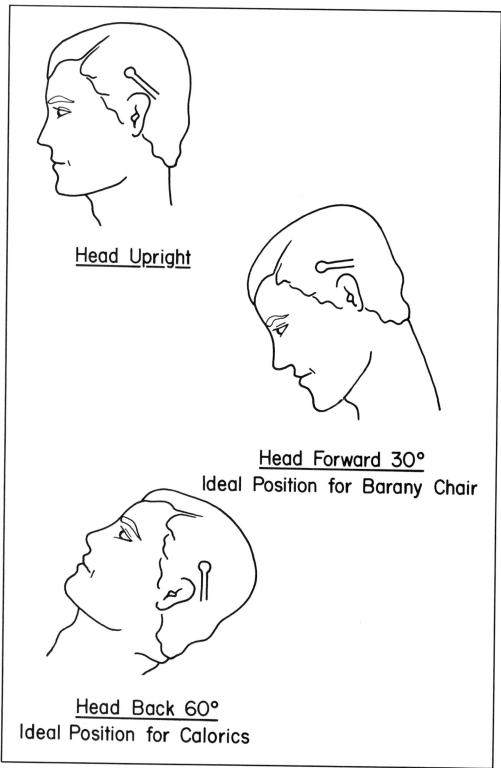

Head Upright

Head Forward 30°
Ideal Position for Barany Chair

Head Back 60°
Ideal Position for Calorics

Fig. 2-3

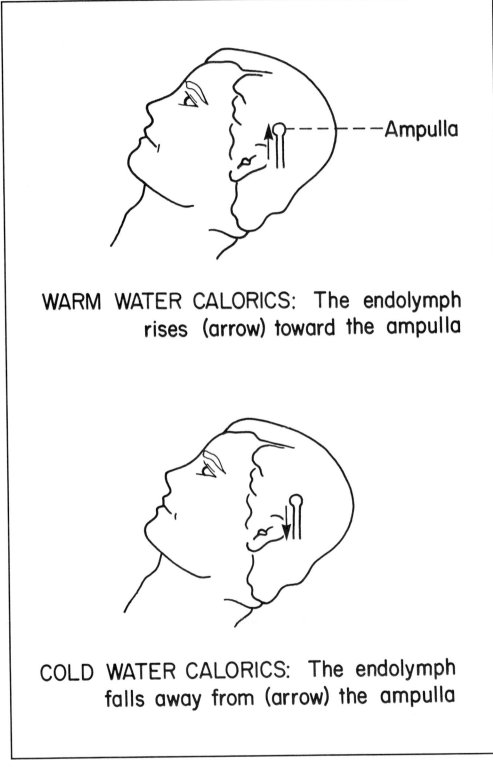

WARM WATER CALORICS: The endolymph rises (arrow) toward the ampulla

COLD WATER CALORICS: The endolymph falls away from (arrow) the ampulla

Fig. 2-4

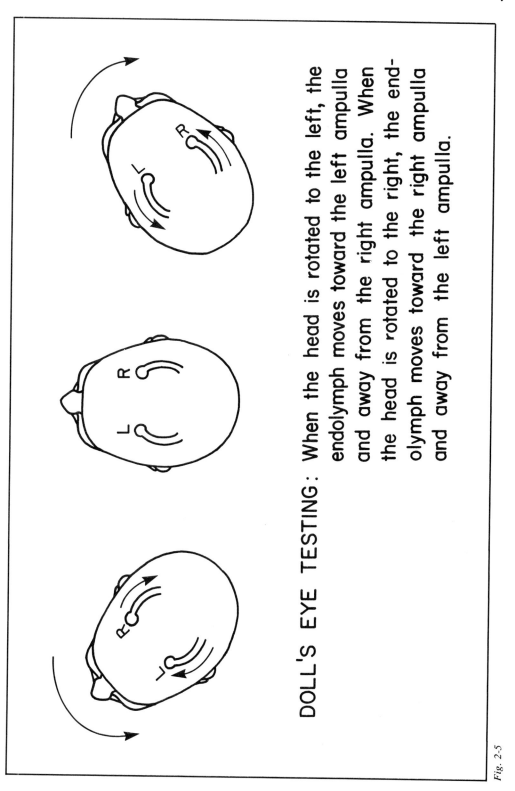

DOLL'S EYE TESTING: When the head is rotated to the left, the endolymph moves toward the left ampulla and away from the right ampulla. When the head is rotated to the right, the endolymph moves toward the right ampulla and away from the left ampulla.

Fig. 2-5

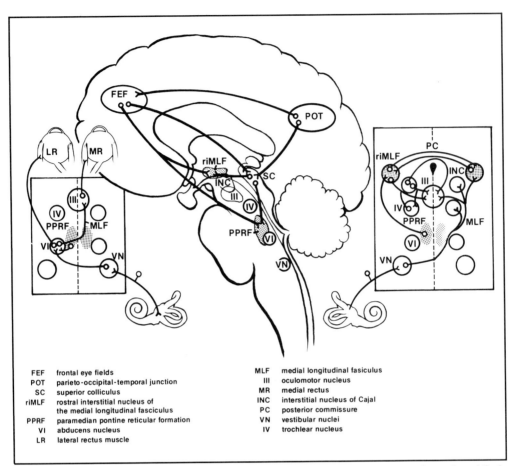

Fig. 2-6. Summary of eye movement control. Center: FEF and SC are involved in the production of saccades, while the POT is important in the production of pursuit. Left: Brainstem pathways for horizontal gaze. Axons from cell bodies in PPRF travel to ipsilateral VI where they synapse with abducens motoneurons whose axons travel to ipsilateral LR. Abducens internuclear neurons have axons that cross the midline and travel in the MLF to III, specifically MR subnucleus (in contralateral eye). Right: Brainstem pathways for vertical gaze. Commands from the riMLF for upward saccades pass through PC, while commands for downward saccades project caudally to III and IV. (Reprinted with permission from Miller NR: Walsh and Hoyt's Clinical Neuro-Ophthalmology. Baltimore, Williams & Wilkins, 1985, Vol. 2, p. 627).

    b. Stimuli

        1) Disparity between the location of images on the retina of each eye. This leads to fusional vergence

        2) Loss of focus of images on the retina (retinal blur). This leads to accommodative vergence

    c. Vergence movements occur as a synkinesis with accommodation of the lens and pupillary constriction (the near triad)

C. Neural pathways for eye movements (Fig. 2-6)

    1. FEM: saccades

        a. Mediated by parallel pathways that converge in the brainstem from

            1) frontal eye fields (Fronto-Mesencephalic pathways)

            2) superior colliculus

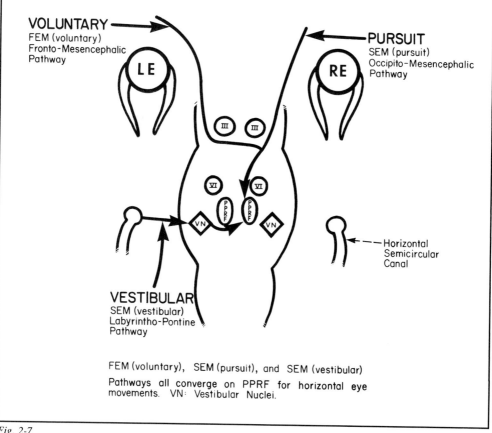

VOLUNTARY
FEM (voluntary)
Fronto-Mesencephalic
Pathway

LE

RE

PURSUIT
SEM (pursuit)
Occipito-Mesencephalic
Pathway

Horizontal
Semicircular
Canal

VESTIBULAR
SEM (vestibular)
Labyrintho-Pontine
Pathway

FEM (voluntary), SEM (pursuit), and SEM (vestibular)
Pathways all converge on PPRF for horizontal eye
movements. VN: Vestibular Nuclei.

Fig. 2-7

b. Fronto-Mesencephalic pathways originate in area 8 of the frontal lobe and course dorsomedially to pass through the anterior limb of the internal capsule, through the thalamus to decussate in the lower midbrain and upper pons and terminate in the PPRF (Paramedian Pontine Reticular Formation) in the lower pons (Fig. 2-7)

c. Stimulation of the left area 8 results in conjugate movement of the eyes to the right side

d. Stimulation of the right area 8 results in conjugate movement of the eyes to the left side

e. Collicular pathways appear to originate in the ventral portions of the superior colliculus and have an effect on the contralateral PPRF

2. FEM: nystagmus quick phases

a. Originate in paramedian reticular formation of the pons and midbrain

b. This phylogenetically old quick-phase system appears to share the same anatomic substrate as the newer voluntary FEM system

3. SEM: smooth pursuit (Parieto-Occipito-Temporal-Mesencephalic pathway)

a. General agreement that the parieto-occipito-temporal junction is an important structure in the cortical control of smooth pursuit

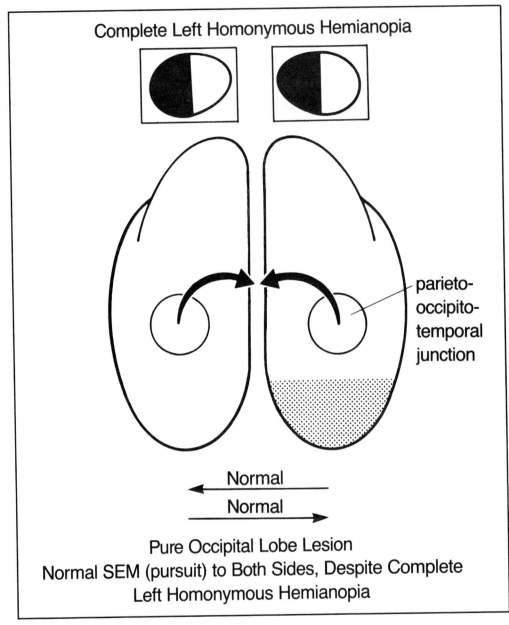

Complete Left Homonymous Hemianopia

parieto-
occipito-
temporal
junction

Normal

Normal

Pure Occipital Lobe Lesion
Normal SEM (pursuit) to Both Sides, Despite Complete
Left Homonymous Hemianopia

Fig. 2-8

    b. Pathways that transmit pursuit commands to the brainstem and cerebellum
       are incompletely understood (Fig. 2-6)
    c. Clinically, this system is best understood in terms of ipsilateral control: the
       right parieto-occipito-temporal junction controls smooth pursuit to the
       right, and the left junction to the left
    d. A pure occipital lobe lesion, despite the production of a homonymous
       hemianopia, will not cause deficiency of pursuit eye movements, since the

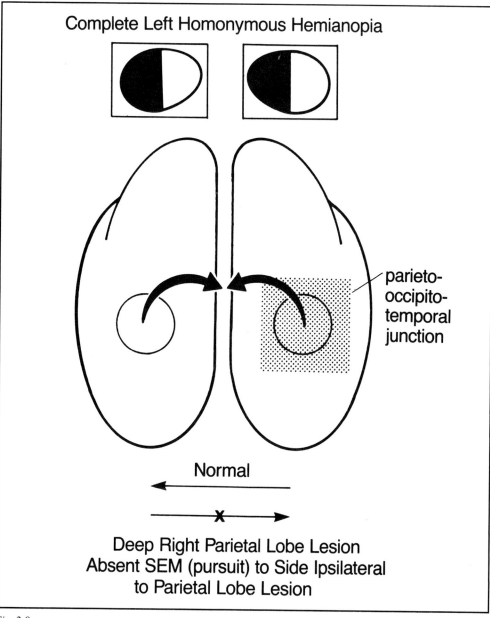

Fig. 2-9

pursuit pathways remain intact (Fig. 2-8)

e. Once the half-macula (of the remaining visual field) is able to achieve fixation, the eye is able to pursue the target to either side

f. General rule: patients with homonymous hemianopia due to optic tract, temporal lobe, or occipital lobe lesions will not have difficulty with smooth pursuit to either side

g. Deep parietal lobe lesions disrupt optomotor fibers intended for the ipsilat-

53

eral pons and thereby disrupt smooth pursuit to the ipsilateral side; the patient may still be able to pursue a target to the side ipsilateral of the lesion, but it will be admixed with catch-up FEM, thus exhibiting non-smooth, cog-wheel pursuit (Fig. 2-9)

    h. Deep parietal lobe lesions result in asymmetric OKN with decreased OKN response when the drum is rotated toward the side of the lesion (see Chapter 1)

4. SEM: optokinetic

    a. Serves as a means of image stabilization to supplement the fading vestibular response of sustained head rotation

    b. OKN ensures clear, stable vision and an appropriate perception of motion both during and after head rotation

    c. Pathways unknown, but thought (based on animal experimentation) that visual stimuli project via brainstem pathways to sum with labyrinthine signals in the vestibular nuclei

5. SEM: vestibular (Labyrinthine-Pontine pathway)

    a. Information from the ampulla of the right horizontal semicircular canal is delivered to the left horizontal gaze center, resulting in SEM (vestibular) to the left side

    b. Information from the ampulla of the left horizontal semicircular canal is delivered to the right horizontal gaze center (Fig. 2-7), resulting in SEM (vestibular) to the right side

    c. Information from the anterior and posterior semicircular canals results in combinations of rotary and vertical eye movements; this probably accounts for the horizontal-rotary nystagmus being a hallmark of labyrinthine disease

6. SEM: vergence (Occipito-Mesencephalic pathway)

    a. Disconjugate eye movements enable bifoveal fixation in space from infinity to the near point of convergence

    b. The near synkinesis pathway begins in area 19 and descends to the III nerve nuclei, resulting in accommodation, miosis, and convergence

7. Note, in Figure 2-7, that the voluntary FEM and the vestibular SEM pathways converge on the contralateral PPRF; the pursuit SEM pathway had been traditionally believed to converge on the ipsilateral PPRF. However, recent evidence suggests otherwise. For clinical purposes, few mistakes will be made if the traditional approach is utilized

8. Each PPRF in the lower pons is the beginning of the final common pathway for all ipsilateral conjugate eye movements

9. Regardless of how the information arrives, whether voluntary, by pursuit, or by vestibular stimulus, once it reaches the PPRF, that information will travel by the same final common pathway to eventuate in conjugate movement of the eye to the ipsilateral side

10. Use Figure 2-10 as a reminder of the course of lateralization of the three conjugate eye movement pathways. Two systems (voluntary and vestibular) have contralateral action and one system (pursuit) has ipsilateral action

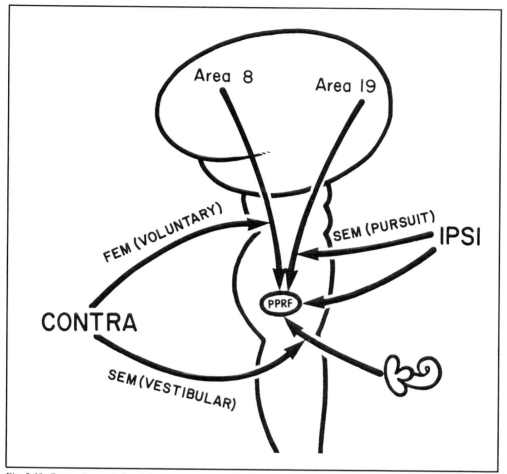

Fig. 2-10. Composite reminder of the course and lateralization of the three conjugate horizontal eye movement pathways.

D. PPRF: Paramedian Pontine Reticular Formation

1. The PPRF serves as the starting point for the final common pathway for conjugate horizontal eye movements
2. PPRF is located just ventral to the medial longitudinal fasciculus and extends from the abducens nucleus to just caudal to the trochlear nucleus
3. PPRF may be referred to as the "horizontal gaze center"
4. Figure 2-11 is a diagrammatic representation of the internuclear connections that make possible the simultaneous contraction of a lateral rectus and its contralateral medial rectus, resulting in conjugate horizontal eye movements
5. The right abducens nucleus is the site of horizontal versional command. The nucleus contains two types of neurons: 1) abducens motoneurons with axons that innervate the ipsilateral lateral rectus; 2) abducens internuclear neurons, with axons that project through the contralateral medial longitudinal fasciculus, to the medial rectus subdivision of the contralateral oculomotor nucleus

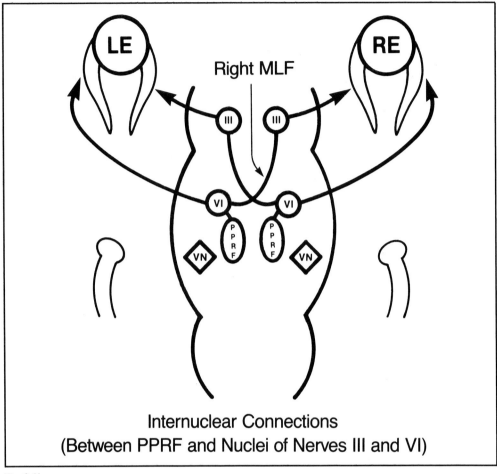

Right MLF

Internuclear Connections
(Between PPRF and Nuclei of Nerves III and VI)

Fig. 2-11

6. The left PPRF sends fibers to the left abducens nucleus, thereby causing left conjugate gaze, while the right PPRF produces right conjugate gaze

E. INO: Internuclear Ophthalmoplegia

1. A lesion of the medial longitudinal fasciculus (MLF) blocks information from the contralateral PPRF to the ipsilateral third nerve nucleus (Fig. 2-12); this "internuclear" lesion results in the clinical phenomenon of an internuclear ophthalmoplegia (INO)

   a. Deficient adduction during attempted conjugate gaze away from the side of the MLF lesion

   b. Abduction nystagmus—i.e., nystagmus of the abducting eye during attempted conjugate gaze away from the side of the lesion

   c. An MLF lesion is on the same side as the eye with the medial rectus (adduction) weakness. INO is named for the side of the MLF lesion

   d. Usually, medial rectus function is intact when convergence is stimulated (Cogan's posterior INO)

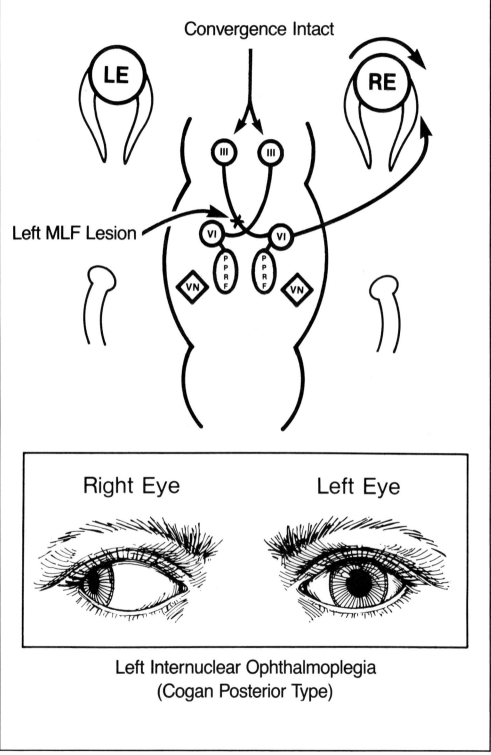

Convergence Intact

LE

RE

Left MLF Lesion

III III

VI VI

P P R F P P R F

VN VN

Right Eye   Left Eye

Left Internuclear Ophthalmoplegia
(Cogan Posterior Type)

Fig. 2-12

57

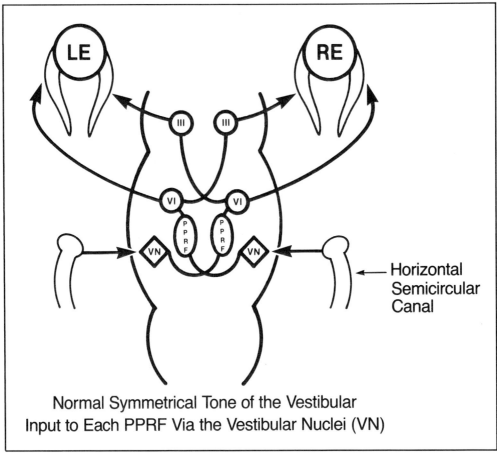

Normal Symmetrical Tone of the Vestibular
Input to Each PPRF Via the Vestibular Nuclei (VN)

Fig. 2-13

    e. INO produced by a mesencephalic lesion is usually bilateral and may have an absence of convergence (Cogan's anterior INO)

    f. Unilateral or bilateral INO in a young adult is most likely due to multiple sclerosis; whereas a unilateral INO in a patient over age 50 is most likely due to brainstem vascular disease

    g. WEBINO (Wall-Eyed Bilateral INO) syndrome refers to an exotropic patient who has bilateral INO's. It is impossible to exclude involvement of the medial rectus subnuclei as well as both MLF's

F. Vestibularly-Elicited Horizontal Eye Movement

    1. Figure 2-13 shows that the horizontal semicircular canals, at rest, deliver an equal amount of innervation to the contralateral PPRF, maintaining a balanced situation for the four horizontal rectus muscles

    2. Noncomatose Patient

        a. When warm water is placed in the right ear, the endolymph moves toward the ampulla of the horizontal canal (Fig. 2-4), causing an increased tone of input received by the left PPRF (Fig. 2-14), thereby resulting in an

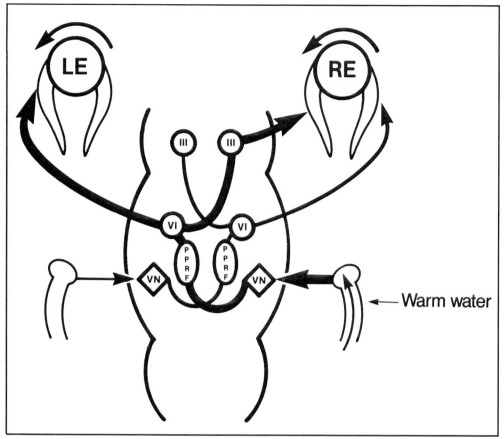

Fig. 2-14. Warm water in the right ear causes shift of endolymph toward the ampulla, thereby increasing the vestibular tone and resulting in a slow movement of the eyes to the left side. The compensatory fast phase will be directed back to the right side (COWS).

increased tone to the left sixth nerve nucleus and right MLF-medial rectus subnucleus, eventuating in slow conjugate contraction (vestibular SEM) of the left lateral rectus muscle and the right medial rectus muscle

b. There will be a compensatory FEM (fast phase) back to the right side, and the combination of left (vestibular) SEM and right (compensatory) FEM produces the clinical phenomenon of right-beating nystagmus following warm water in the right ear

c. Cold water will produce the opposite response, in that endolymph will now move away from the ampulla of the horizontal canal, causing slow conjugate contraction (vestibular SEM) to the ipsilateral side, and a compensatory FEM back to the opposite side (Fig. 2-15)

d. J. Lawton Smith has pointed out the usefulness of the mnemonic of COWS (Cold Opposite; Warm Same) to remind us that, as we have just seen, Warm water in the Right ear results in Right-beating nystagmus; Cold water in the Left ear results in Right-beating nystagmus; Left-beating nystagmus would

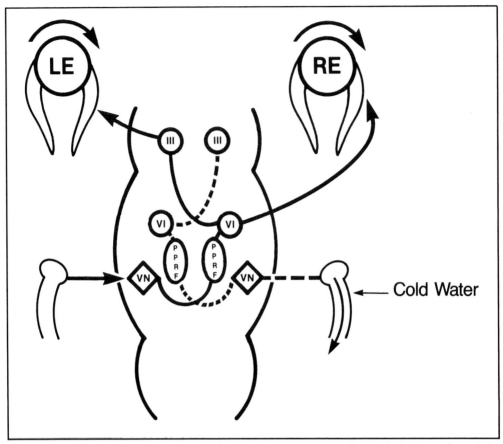

Fig. 2-15. Cold water in the right ear causes shift of endolymph away from the ampulla, thereby decreasing the vestibular tone and allowing the vestibular tone from the left side to be dominant. This results in a slow movement of the eyes to the right. The compensatory fast phase will therefore be directed to the left side (COWS).

        be produced by Cold water in the Right or Warm water in the Left ear

e. However, note (Fig. 2-14) that the vestibular input produced by the warm water in Right ear is responsible, not for the FEM (jerk movement of the nystagmus) back to the right, but only for the initial SEM to the left; the mnemonic of "COWS" refers to direction of the jerk-component of the calorically-induced nystagmus

f. The FEM (jerk-component) is actually a compensatory (probably fronto-mesencephalic) saccadic movement that is seen only in the noncomatose patient, who has intact fronto-mesencephalic connections

g. Rotational testing for eye movement function in neonates is helpful in determining the state of brainstem pathways for conjugate horizontal gaze

h. Fig. 2-16 illustrates the effect of head rotation on right and left horizontal semicircular canals. The infant's eyes tonically deviate in the direction of the movement, with jerk phase of nystagmus toward the opposite side

3. Comatose Patient

    a. When warm water is placed in the right ear, assuming nuclear and inter-

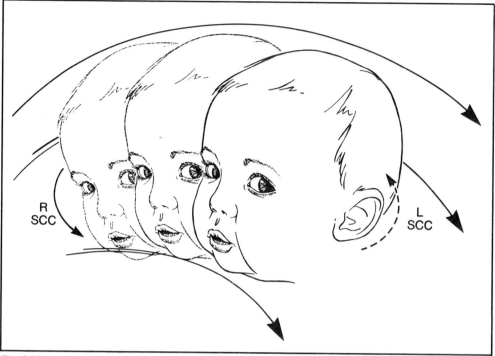

Fig. 2-16. Rotational testing for eye movement function in infants. As infant is spun toward its left (toward examiner's right), the eyes will tonically deviate in the direction of the movement, with jerk phase of nystagmus toward the opposite side. This leads to stimulation of right semicircular canals (SCC) and inhibition of the left SCC.

nuclear brainstem connections are intact, there will be slow tonic conjugate movement (vestibular SEM) of the eyes to the left side, without compensatory right-jerk nystagmus (the fronto-mesencephalic connections are nonfunctional in coma). The eyes will remain deviated to the left side for 30-60 seconds and then return back to the midline as the symmetrical tone of the semicircular canals is reestablished

    b. Similarly, when cold water is placed in the right ear, the patient's eyes will slowly, tonically deviate to the right side, and then return to the midline

4. Doll's eye testing with rotation to the head to the right also produces a tonic SEM (vestibular) to the left; Figure 2-5 illustrates that this results from a combination of shift of the endolymph away from the left ampulla and toward the right ampulla, thereby decreasing the input from the left ampulla and increasing the input from the right ampulla

5. The SEM tone produced by doll's eye testing is not sustained enough to result in compensatory FEM (jerk nystagmus)

G. Vertical Gaze Pathways

1. No "vertical gaze center" has yet been identified, yet certain mesencephalic structures are important for vertical eye movements (Fig. 2-6)

2. The rostral interstitial nucleus of the medial longitudinal fasciculus (riMLF) is necessary in generating vertical saccades. Each nucleus lies dorsomedial to the

red nucleus at the junction of the midbrain and thalamus

3. There appears to be an anatomic separation of cells within the riMLF subserving upgaze and downgaze, but disagreement as to which part is responsible for which function

4. Upgaze: upward saccadic command from the riMLF must pass dorsally through the posterior commissure to the third nerve nuclei

5. Downgaze: downgaze saccade command projects dorsally and caudally to the third and fourth cranial nerve nuclei

6. Each riMLF receives descending projections from the frontal eye fields, and ascending projections from the vestibular nuclei and PPRF

H. Horizontal Gaze Abnormalities

1. Supranuclear
   a. Acute cerebrovascular accident (CVA) affecting frontal lobe (area 8)
      1) Eyes (and usually head) tonically deviate toward the side of the lesion, since the contralateral area 8 has unopposed action
      2) Doll's eye testing and calorics can turn the eyes contralateral to the lesion (since the SEM [vestibular] pathway is intact), but the eyes then return to tonic deviation toward the lesion
      3) Within three to seven days the patients begin to exhibit voluntary eye movements away from the lesion
   b. Congenital ocular motor apraxia
      1) Deficiency of voluntary horizontal eye movements
      2) Vertical movements normal; horizontal SEM (vestibular) normal
      3) Random saccades and pursuit horizontal eye movements may be seen
      4) When the patient seeks to change visual fixation horizontally, he does so by "thrusting" his head toward the desired direction of gaze
      5) The head movement elicits a contralateral SEM (vestibular), thereby neutralizing some of the change in gaze-direction accomplished with the head movement
      6) Therefore, the patient demonstrates an over-shoot (of the target) with the head movement in order to overcome a counteracting SEM (vestibular) and thereby fixate on the new target
      7) The patient then straightens his head while maintaining fixation on the new target
      8) The head movement and "over-shoot" produce the phenomenon of head thrusting, which the hallmark of congenital ocular motor apraxia
      9) The head-thrusting becomes less prominent with age
      10) Congenital ocular motor apraxia may be associated with developmental CNS defects including Gaucher's disease, spinocerebellar degeneration and mental retardation
   c. Balint's syndrome: acquired ocular motor apraxia
      1) Patients with extensive bilateral cerebral disease (parieto-occipital)
      2) Demonstrate absence of FEM (voluntary) and SEM (pursuit) in all directions, with intact SEM (vestibular) and intact random eye movements

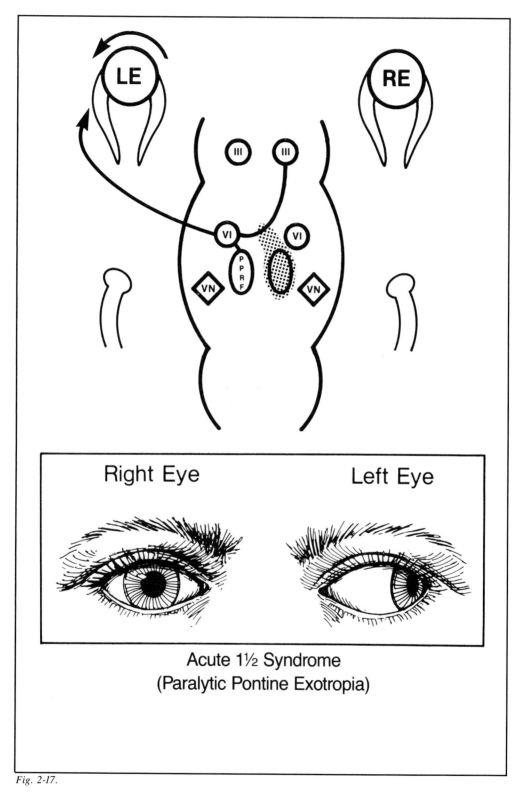

Acute 1½ Syndrome
(Paralytic Pontine Exotropia)

Fig. 2-17.

3) Frequently have dementia and visual field defects

d. Spasticity of conjugate gaze (Cogan's sign)

    1) A "screening" test for cerebral disease

    2) Normally, during forced lid closure, each eye is deviated super-olaterally (Bell's phenomenon)

    3) Patients with lesions of the temporal or parietal lobe may show conjugate deviation of the eye superiorly and away from the side of the lesion

    4) This spasticity of conjugate gaze is not seen with frontal lobe lesions, except during the acute phase when the eye is tonically deviated toward the lesion (see I.1.a, above)

    5) Cogan's sign is of lateralizing but not localizing value

2. Pontine conjugate gaze palsy (PPRF lesion)

    a. Unilateral PPRF lesion creates an ipsilateral conjugate horizontal gaze palsy

    b. With acute lesions, the eyes may be deviated contralaterally

    c. Ipsilaterally directed saccades and quick phases of nystagmus are small and slow and do not carry the eyes past the midline

    d. Smooth pursuit and slow phases of OKN may be preserved, in both directions, within the intact field of movement, but cannot bring the eyes past the midline

    e. In some patients vestibular stimuli (e.g. calorics) drive the eyes across the midline. Presumably, the ipsilateral abducens nucleus and its direct vestibular input are intact, and the PPRF lesion is more rostral

3. Internuclear ophthalmoplegia—see section E (above)

√4. One-and-a-half syndrome

    a. Lesion of the PPRF and ipsilateral MLF (Fig. 2-17)

    b. Pontine conjugate gaze palsy to the ipsilateral side ("one")

    c. INO on gaze to the contralateral side (the "half")

√5. Paralytic pontine exotropia

    a. A transient phenomenon seen in the one-and-a-half syndrome during the first few days after onset

    b. The PPRF lesion causes the contralateral PPRF to be unopposed; therefore, the eyes tend to deviate conjugately away from the lesion

    c. However, because of the INO, the ipsilateral eye cannot adduct

    d. The eye contralateral to the MLF lesion remains tonically abducted and demonstrates an exotropia

I. Vertical Gaze Abnormalities

1. Downgaze palsy—due to midbrain disease (stroke, tumor) with lesions involving the riMLF just rostral to the third nerve nucleus and dorsomedially to the red nucleus

2. Upgaze palsy—association with lesions located more dorsally, contiguous with the posterior commissure

3. Dorsal midbrain syndrome

    a. Also known as "pretectal syndrome," "Sylvian aqueduct syndrome," or "Parinaud's syndrome"

  b. Supranuclear paresis of vertical gaze: vertical FEM (voluntary) and SEM (pursuit) are affected, but vertical SEM (vestibular) is intact
  c. Other associated eye signs
    1) Light-near dissociation of the pupils
    2) Convergence-retraction nystagmus
    3) Lid retraction (Collier's sign)
    4) Spasm/paresis of convergence
    5) Spasm/paresis of accommodation
    6) Skew deviation (see Section K below)
4. Monocular elevation paresis
  a. No abnormality in primary position or looking down, but diplopia in upgaze due to limitation of elevation in one eye
  b. Associated pupillary abnormality which may include anisocoria, sluggish light reaction, and light-near dissociation
  c. Forced ductions and Tensilon testing are both negative
  d. Presumed interruption of supranuclear input from riMLF (mediating upgaze) to third nerve nucleus
5. Progressive Supranuclear Palsy
  a. Steele-Richardson-Olszewski syndrome
  b. Progressive conjugate paresis of gaze in all directions, but usually affecting vertical gaze (especially downgaze) initially
  c. SEM (vestibular) better than FEM (voluntary) and SEM (pursuit)
  d. Some clinical features similar to Parkinsonism
    1) Nuchal rigidity
    2) Seborrheic skin changes
    3) Usually no testing tremor
  e. Progressive dementia and death usually within five years
6. Oculogyric crisis
  a. Tonic vertical supranuclear deviation of the eyes; able to overcome with SEM (vestibular) but eyes then return to the tonically deviated position
  b. Seen with post-encephalitic Parkinsonism and phenothiazine toxicity

J. Skew Deviation
1. An acquired vertical ocular deviation resulting from supranuclear dysfunction
2. May be comitant or noncomitant
3. May be seen with INO and/or gaze-evoked vertical nystagmus
4. Implicates brainstem or cerebellar disease, but otherwise has no localizing value

Bibliography

BOOKS

Gay AJ, Newman NM, Keltner JL et al: Eye Movement Disorders. St. Louis, CV Mosby, 1974.

Leigh RJ, Zee DS: The Neurology of Eye Movement. Philadelphia, FA Davis Co., 1983.

Smith JL: Optokinetic nystagmus: its use in topical neuroophthalmologic diagnosis. Springfield, CC Thomas, 1963.

CHAPTERS

Daroff RB, Troost BT: Supranuclear disorders of eye movements, in Duane, TD (ed): Clinical Ophthalmology. Hagerstown, Harper & Row, 1978, Vol. 2, Chap. 10, In press.

Miller NR: Walsh and Hoyt's Clinical Neuro-Ophthalmology. Baltimore, Williams & Wilkins, 1985, Chapters 32-35, pp. 559-784.

ARTICLES

Bloedel JR: The physiologic basis of conjugate eye movements. Am J Otol (Suppl.) 1985; 6:35-38.

Cogan DG: Congenital ocular motor apraxia. Can J Ophthalmol 1966; 1:253-260.

Cogan DG: Internuclear ophthalmoplegia: typical and atypical. Arch Ophthalmol 1970; 84:583-589.

Cogan DG: Paralysis of down-gaze. Arch Ophthalmol 1974; 91:192-199.

Fisher CM: Some neuro-ophthalmological observations. J Neurol Neurosurg Psychiatry 1967; 30:383-392.

Hatcher MA, Klintworth GK: The Sylvian aqueduct syndrome. Arch Neurol 1966; 15:215-222.

Jampel RS, Fells P: Monocular elevation paresis caused by a central nervous system lesion. Arch Ophthalmol 1968; 80:45-57.

Keane JR: Ocular skew deviation. Arch Neurol 1975; 32:185-190.

Pola J, Robinson DA: An explanation of eye movements seen in internuclear ophthalmoplegia. 1976; 33:447-452.

Sharpe JA, Rosenberg MA, Hoyt WF, et al: Paralytic pontine exotropia. Neurology 1974; 24:1076-1081.

Smith JL, Gay AJ, Cogan DG: The spasticity of conjugate gaze phenomenon. Arch Ophthalmol 1959; 62:694-696.

Smith JL, Ziepen I, Gay AJ, et al: Nystagmus retractorius. Arch Ophthalmol 1959; 62:864-867.

Steele JC, Richarson JC, Olszewski J: Progressive supranuclear palsy: A heterogeneous degeneration involving the brain stem, basal ganglia and cerebellum with vertical gaze and pseudobulbar palsy, nuchal dystonia and dementia. Arch Neurol 1964; 1:333-359.

Trojanowski JQ, Wray SH: Vertical gaze ophthalmoplegia: selective paralysis of downgaze. Neurology 1980; 30:605-610.

3

Nystagmus and Related Ocular Oscillations

A. Definition: Rhythmic, involuntary to-and-fro oscillation of the eyes
B. Nystagmus jargon
   1. Type
      a. Pendular: phases of equal velocity
      b. Jerk: phases of unequal velocity
   2. Direction: the direction of the fast component
   3. Plane: horizontal, vertical, diagonal, rotary, circular, elliptical
   4. Amplitude: fine, medium, coarse
   5. Rate: rapid, slow
   6. Conjugacy: conjugate if both eyes demonstrate same movement; dissociated if the eyes have different movements (e.g. one eye has horizontal nystagmus and the other circular; or one eye has a large amplitude or a faster rate of nystagmus
   7. Alexander's law: jerk nystagmus usually increases in amplitude with gaze in the direction of the fast phase
   8. Null zone: that field of gaze in which the nystagmus intensity is minimal
   9. Neutral zone: that field of gaze in which bilateral jerk nystagmus reverses direction
C. Congenital nystagmus and afferent visual system disorders
   1. Traditional description of two forms of congenital nystagmus
      a. Afferent nystagmus—nystagmus due to poor vision
      b. Efferent nystagmus—nystagmus due to ocular motor disturbance
   2. Causes of poor vision early in life include
      a. Ocular albinism
      b. Aniridia
      c. Achromatopsia
      d. Congenital optic nerve disease: atrophy, hypoplasia
      e. Congenital cataracts
   3. On the basis of eye movement recordings, congenital nystagmus associated with poor visual function cannot be distinguished from congenital nystagmus without afferent visual system dysfunction
   4. Therefore, congenital nystagmus is conceptualized as a motor disturbance of ocular motility
   5. Nystagmus secondary to visual loss can only be diagnosed if it is known that

the nystagmus developed after the visual problem began. Otherwise, the nystagmus may coexist with the visual disturbance, but a causal relationship cannot be assumed

D. Clinical classification of nystagmus

1. Physiologic nystagmus
2. Specific, recognizable, localizing types of nystagmus: eleven types of nystagmus that have specific diagnostic, clinical value
3. Nonspecific, nonlocalizing gaze-evoked nystagmus
4. Related oscillations

E. Physiologic nystagmus

1. End-position nystagmus—three forms
    a. Fatigue nystagmus: occurs after prolonged ($>$ 10-15 seconds) deviation of eyes
    b. Unsustained end-position nystagmus: seen initially at extremes of gaze (except downgaze) but resolves in five to ten seconds
    c. Sustained end-position nystagmus: symmetric, fine nystagmus in extreme right and left gaze; disappears when gaze returned 15-20° back toward primary position
2. Optokinetic nystagmus (OKN)
    a. Can be conceptualized simplistically as a combination of SEM (pursuit) and compensatory FEM (saccade) to pick up fixation of the next target on the OKN stimulus
    b. OKN is abnormal when it is "asymmetric": greater OKN demonstrated when target is moving in one direction compared to the opposite
    c. Asymmetric OKN (diminished OKN when targets moving toward side of the lesion) may be seen in association with homonymous hemianopia due to a deep parietal lesion (see Chapters 1 and 2)
    d. However, a homonymous hemianopia alone does not cause the diminished OKN; normal OKN seen in a patient with hemianopia due to optic tract, temporal lobe, and occipital lobe lesions
    e. OKN test of vision: can substantiate the presence of vision in a patient with psychogenic blindness
3. Caloric nystagmus (see Chapter 2)
    a. Combination of SEM (vestibular) and compensatory FEM saccade
    b. Vestibular SEM elicited by stimulation (shift of endolymph toward ampulla) or inhibition (shift of endolymph away from ampulla) of one or more semicircular canals
    c. Unilateral irrigation produces nystagmus which is either horizontal, rotary, or oblique, depending on the position of the head
    d. Bilateral simultaneous caloric stimulation produces vertical nystagmus: CUWD (cold, up; warm, down; direction of fast phase of nystagmus)
4. Rotational nystagmus (see Fig. 2-5)
    a. Rotating or accelerating head movements induce movement of endolymph in the semicircular canals which results in jerk nystagmus
    b. During rotation, nystagmus fast phases in the direction of the rotation

    c. Following cessation of rotation, the post rotary nystagmus is oppositely directed

    d. Useful in the evaluation of the ocular motor system in infants (Fig. 2-16)

F. Specific, recognizable, localizing types of nystagmus

  1. Congenital nystagmus

    a. Includes all forms of nystagmus noted at birth or within the perinatal period

    b. Congenital nystagmus is usually of horizontal form, but may be vertical, circular, or elliptical; it may be pendular or jerk

    c. Daroff lists eleven characteristics of congenital nystagmus

       1) binocular and associated

       2) similar amplitude in both eyes

       3) no oscillopsia (illusion of environmental movement)

       4) abolished in sleep

       5) may have associated head oscillation

       6) dampened by convergence

       7) increased by fixation effort

       8) may have superimposed latent nystagmus (see below)

       9) inversion of the optokinetic reflex, i.e. induced nystagmus in the opposite direction to that expected

      10) distinctive wave forms with eye movement recording: increasing velocity exponential of the slow phase

      11) uniplanar: hallmark of congenital nystagmus. Plane of the nystagmus, usually horizontal, remains unchanged in all positions of gaze including vertical gaze. This phenomenon is seen in only three entities

        a) congenital nystagmus

        b) peripheral vestibular nystagmus

        c) periodic alternating nystagmus

    d. Can frequently identify a "null zone" of gaze in which the nystagmus is least marked and the visual acuity is best

    e. Patient may manifest head turn to keep the eyes in a null zone; may require muscle surgery (Kestenbaum procedure) in order to place the null zone in the primary position

    f. High astigmatism frequently found

    g. Nystagmus is usually dampened by convergence, so the patient usually has good near acuity and can do well in school

    h. Patients may be helped by contact lenses to correct the astigmatism and obviate the visual aberrations created by an eye wiggling behind a spectacle lens which has a high astigmatic correction

    i. Patients may also be helped by base-out prism glasses that induce convergence (with its nystagmus-dampening effect) during distance fixation

  2. Latent nystagmus

    a. Nystagmus seen only when one eye is covered

    b. The patient develops bilateral jerk nystagmus with the jerk component directed away from the covered eye

    c. Visual acuity diminished (due to nystagmus) when each eye is tested

separately; acuity improves when both eyes are uncovered
    d. May coexist with ongoing primary position pendular, jerk or rotary nystagmus which converts to latent nystagmus pattern following monocular occlusion
    e. This type of nystagmus is congenital and may be seen in association with dissociated vertical deviation and strabismus (usually esotropia)

3. Spasmus nutans
    a. Triad of head turn, head nodding, and nystagmus
    b. Begins in first 18 months of life and resolves by three years of age
    c. Horizontal or vertical, pendular, low-amplitude, high-frequency nystagmus
    d. May be unilateral or of different amplitude in each eye
    e. Acquired monocular nystagmus has been reported in initial sign of anterior visual pathway glioma
    f. Therefore, spasmus nutans is a diagnosis of exclusion requiring high-resolution CT scanning to exclude afferent visual pathway pathology

4. Dissociated nystagmus
    a. The nystagmus in one eye is different than the other
    b. For example, one eye has vertical and the other eye has horizontal nystagmus
    c. Alternatively, one eye demonstrates greater amplitude than the other
    d. Dissociation of the eyes usually indicates posterior fossa disease
    e. The abduction nystagmus of INO is an example of dissociated nystagmus

5. Downbeat nystagmus
    a. Fast phase down, while the eyes are in primary position of gaze; downbeat often seen during lateral gaze
    b. Usually associated with long-standing lesion at the cervicomedullary junction (at the level of the foramen magnum)
        1) Arnold-Chiari malformation
        2) Spinocerebellar degeneration
        3) Brainstem stroke
        4) Multiple sclerosis
        5) Platybasia

6. Upbeat nystagmus
    a. Fast phase up, while the eyes are in primary position of gaze; upbeating during lateral gaze as well
    b. May be of large or small amplitude
    c. Most patients have intrinsic brainstem disease. Some reported cases due to lesion of cerebellar vermis and in many cases location of pathologic lesion is uncertain

7. See-saw nystagmus
    a. Pendular
    b. Conjugate-rotary with disconjugate-vertical component
    c. One eye supraducts and incyclotorts; the other infraducts and excyclotorts
    d. Frequently associated with suprasellar lesions and bitemporal hemianopia
    e. May be congenital

8. Convergence-retraction nystagmus
   a. Jerk convergence-retraction movements due to co-contraction of the extra-ocular muscles, especially on attempted convergence or upward gaze
   b. Dorsal midbrain syndrome (Sylvian aqueduct, pretectal, Parinaud's syndrome)
      1) Defective vertical gaze, especially upward
      2) Light-near dissociation of the pupils
      3) Lid retraction (Collier's sign)
      4) Convergence-retraction nystagmus
      5) Spasm/paresis of convergence
      6) Spasm/paresis of accommodation
      7) Skew deviation
   c. The convergence-retraction nystagmus is best seen during testing of the eyes with down-going OKN targets, which require upward saccades
   d. J. Lawton Smith's age-differential of possible etiologies:
      0 (infant): congenital aqueductal stenosis
      10-year-old: pinealoma
      20-year-old: head trauma
      30-year-old: brainstem vascular malformation
      40-year-old: long-standing multiple sclerosis
      50-year-old: basilar artery stroke
9. Periodic alternating nystagmus
   a. Jerk nystagmus, while eyes in primary position, with the fast component to one side for 60-90 seconds, followed by 3-5 seconds rest period of little or no nystagmus, then slowly leading to a crescendo-decrescendo of fast-component to the other side, lasting 60-90 seconds, followed by a 3-5 second rest period
   b. This cycle repeats continuously
   c. Nystagmus remains horizontal in vertical gaze
   d. Etiologies
      1) Congenital
      2) Vestibulo-cerebellar disease: stroke, multiple sclerosis, spinocerebellar degeneration
      3) Severe, acquired bilateral visual loss (optic atrophy, vitreous hemorrhage)
   e. Some patients have responded to treatment with baclofen with disappearance of their periodic alternating nystagmus
   f. Correction of visual loss (vitrectomy) may abolish nystagmus
10. Vestibular nystagmus
   a. Due to dysfunction of vestibular end-organ, nerve, or nuclear complex
   b. Usually a horizontal-rotary or purely horizontal, primary position jerk nystagmus
   c. Peripheral vestibular nystagmus
      1) Nystagmus characteristics
         a) Unidirectional

        b) Nystagmus of greatest amplitude when gaze in direction of the fast component (Alexander's law)

        c) Invariably has a rotary component

        d) Uniplanar

    2) Fast phase beats away from the diseased end-organ

    3) Frequently associated with vertigo, tinnitus, deafness

    4) Labyrinthine disease usually causes suppression of labyrinthine input, thereby stimulating the symptoms caused by cold water calorics; thus, cold water in the left ear of a normal subject reproduces the symptoms of left labyrinthine disease

        a) Nystagmus fast-phase to right (COWS)

        b) The slow component is to the left; therefore, the environment appears to move to the right

        c) The subject past-points to the left

        d) Romberg fall to the left when head in primary position; Romberg fall backwards when the face is turned to the left; Romberg fall forwards when face is turned to the right

    5) Etiologies

        a) Labyrinthitis

        b) Neuronitis

        c) Vascular ischemia

        d) Traumatic

        e) Toxic

  d. Central vestibular nystagmus

    1) Nystagmus characteristics

        a) Unidirectional or bidirectional

        b) May be purely horizontal, or less frequently purely vertical or rotary

        c) Jerk nystagmus may change direction with change in direction of gaze

    2) Vertigo, tinnitus, deafness are usually less prominent symptoms

    3) Romberg direction of fall does not vary with change in head position

    4) Etiology: bilateral brainstem dysfunction due to

        a) Tumor

        b) Trauma

        c) Stroke

        d) Demyelination

11. Voluntary nystagmus

  a. Rapid, low-amplitude, horizontal pendular nystagmus; consists of back-to-back saccades

  b. Patient unable to sustain this type of nystagmus (duration usually less than 30 seconds)

  c. Frequent blinking and closing of eyes

  d. Can stop nystagmus momentarily by having patient change direction of gaze

e. Seen in hysterical patients, malingerers

G. Nonspecific, nonlocalizing, gaze-evoked nystagmus

1. No nystagmus in primary position of gaze
    a. The eleven specific types of nystagmus described above are generally seen while the eyes are in the primary position
    b. The patients with nonspecific gaze-evoked nystagmus demonstrate no nystagmus in the primary position and show nystagmus only during eccentric gaze
        1) Left-jerk nystagmus on gaze left
        2) Right-jerk nystagmus on gaze right
        3) Upbeating nystagmus on gaze up
        4) Downbeating nystagmus on gaze down
2. Downbeating nystagmus seen in gaze down in the patient with nonspecific gaze-evoked nystagmus does not qualify as, and does not have the clinical significance of, "downbeat nystagmus" (see section 5, above)
3. The upbeating nystagmus seen in gaze up in the patient with nonspecific, gaze-evoked nystagmus does not qualify as, and does not have the clinical significance of "upbeat nystagmus" (see section 6, above)
4. Nonspecific gaze-evoked nystagmus has two main etiologies
    a. Drug induced: anticonvulsants (Dilantin, phenobarbital) or any kind of tranquilizer or sedative
    b. Posterior fossa disease: bilateral brainstem and/or cerebellar dysfunction (tumor, trauma, demyelination, vascular infarction) but is of no further localizing value

H. Cerebellar system disease

1. Cardinal cerebellar eye signs
    a. Square wave jerks
    b. Ocular dysmetria
    c. Ocular flutter
    d. Opsoclonus
    e. Nystagmus
        1) Horizontal gaze-evoked; gaze-paretic
        2) Rebound
    f. Ocular myoclonus
    g. Skew deviation
2. Square wave jerks
    a. "Fixation instability": nonrhythmic break in fixation followed by a single movement of refoveation
    b. Square wave jerks are subtle (amplitude 0.5°-3°; latency to refixation, 200 msec); macro-square wave jerks are quite easily seen (amplitude, 4-30°; latency to refixation, 50-150 msec)
    c. So named because of rectangular appearance on eye movement recordings
3. Ocular dysmetria
    a. The ocular equivalent of extremity "past-pointing"

    b. Conjugate hypermetric (overshoot) eye movements during voluntary change of gaze

    c. Patients with ocular dysmetria frequently have cerebellar disease and nystagmus on eccentric gaze; therefore, dysmetria is most reliably detected during refixation back to the primary position

    d. During refixation back to the primary position, the eyes will demonstrate their hypermetria, followed by several oscillations about the new fixation point before the eyes come to rest

    e. A single overshoot with corrective saccades is seen at times in the normal subject during small-amplitude saccade testing

4. Ocular flutter

    a. Spontaneous intermittent bursts of three or four conjugate horizontal micro-oscillations while the patient is maintaining fixation in the primary position

    b. They are like the micro-oscillations (described above) seen after a dysmetric refixation movement, except that ocular flutter occurs spontaneously in the primary position

    c. Patients with ocular flutter usually also demonstrate ocular dysmetria

5. Opsoclonus

    a. Rapid, involuntary, multivectorial (horizontal, vertical, diagonal), unpredictable (chaotic), conjugate fast eye movements that stop during sleep

    b. Also referred to as "saccadomania"

    c. Infants

        1) Neuroblastoma: opsoclonus is a nonmetastatic, distant cerebellar effect seen in association with ataxia and myoclonus, and referred to as the syndrome of "dancing eyes and dancing feet"

        2) Infants may also present with opsoclonus that appears due to an autoimmune disturbance which is responsive to ACTH

    d. Infants and adults: opsoclonus may be seen as a benign, self-limited ocular phenomenon following an infectious encephalopathy

    e. Adults: opsoclonus may be a remote effect of a visceral carcinoma

6. Gaze-evoked and gaze-paretic nystagmus

    a. Most common cause of bidirectional gaze-evoked nystagmus is anticonvulsant or sedative medication

    b. In the absence of drugs, gaze-evoked nystagmus indicates bilateral brainstem and/or cerebellar dysfunction

    c. Gaze-paretic refers to one particular type of gaze-evoked nystagmus which is frequently associated with cerebellar disease

        1) slow rate (1-2 beats/second)

        2) large amplitude

        3) thought due to defective gaze-holding mechanism

        4) patients recovering from a gaze palsy pass through a stage of gaze-paretic nystagmus

7. Rebound nystagmus

    a. Horizontal jerk nystagmus may be detected as

        1) Gaze-evoked nystagmus that will slowly fatigue and be followed by

development of jerk nystagmus in the opposite direction, that is, fast phase toward the primary position

    2) Jerk nystagmus that transiently occurs when the eyes are returned to the primary position following sustained eccentric gaze. The nystagmus has its fast phase in the direction opposite to the sustained deviation

8. Ocular myoclonus
    a. Usually vertical-pendular nystagmus at a rate of 100-150/minute
    b. Synchronous contraction of the face, palate, pharynx, diaphragm, extremity
    c. Caused by a lesion in the "myoclonic triangle," the triangle connecting the following anatomic sites
        1) Red nucleus
        2) Ipsilateral inferior olive
        3) Contralateral dentate nucleus
    d. These movements persist during sleep
9. Skew Deviation (see Chapter 2)

I. Related ocular oscillations

1. Ocular bobbing
    a. Fast, conjugate, downward movement of the eye followed by a slow drift back up to the primary position; just like watching a "bobber" on the water as a fish is nibbling at the bait
    b. The patient is usually comatose and has a massive pontine lesion such as a hemorrhage, infarct, or malignant tumor
    c. May be seen with obstructive hydrocephalus or metabolic encephalopathy
    d. Usually demonstrates no spontaneous or reflex (doll's eye, calorics) horizontal eye movements

2. Superior Oblique Myokymia
    a. See Chapter 6 (section H)

Bibliography

BOOKS

Leigh RJ, Zee DS: The Neurology of Eye Movement. Philadelphia, FA Davis Co., 1982.
Smith JL: Optokinetic nystagmus: its use in topical neuro-ophthalmologic diagnosis. Springfield, CC Thomas, 1963.

CHAPTERS

Burde RM, Savino PJ, Trobe JD: Clinical Decisions in Neuroophthalmology. St. Louis, CV Mosby, 1985, Chapter 6, pp. 197-220.
Dell'Osso LF, Daroff RB, Troost BT: Nystagmus and saccadic intrusions and oscillation. In Duane TD (ed): Clinical Ophthalmology. Hagerstown, Harper & Row, 1978, Vol. 2, Chapter 11, In press.
Miller NR: Walsh and Hoyt's Clinical Neuro-ophthalmology. Baltimore, Williams & Wilkins, 1985, Chapter 37, pp. 892-931.

ARTICLES

Antony JH, Ouvria RA, Wise G: Spasmus nutans—a mistaken identity. Arch Neurol 1980; 37:373-375.
Baloh RW, Honrubia V, Konrad HR: Periodic alternating nystagmus. Brain 1976; 99:11-26.

Baloh RW, Spooner JW: Downbeat nystagmus: a type of central vestibular nystagmus. Neurology 1981; 31:304-310.

Bosch EP, Kennedy SS, Aschenbrener CA: Ocular bobbing: The myth of its localizing value. Neurology 1975; 25:949-953.

Brandt S, Carlsen N, Glentin P, et al: Encephalopathia myoclonica infantalis (Kinsbourne) and neuroblastoma in children. A report of three cases. Dev Med Child Neurol 1974; 16:286-294.

Cogan DG: Congenital nystagmus. Can J Ophthalmol 1967; 2:4-10.

Cogan DG: Dissociated nystagmus with lesions in the posterior fossa. Arch Ophthalmol 1963; 70:361-368.

Cogan DG: Downbeat nystagmus. Arch Ophthalmol 1968; 80:757-768.

Cogan DG: Ocular dysmetria, flutter-like oscillations of the eyes, and opsoclonus. Arch Ophthalmol 1954; 51:318-335.

Davis DG, Smith JL: Periodic alternating nystagmus. Am J Ophthalmol 1971; 72:757-762.

Daroff RB: See-saw nystagmus. Neurology 1965; 15:874-877.

Daroff RB, Troost BT: Upbeat nystagmus. JAMA 1973; 225-312.

Dell'Osso LF, Schmidt D, Daroff RB: Latent, manifest latent, and congenital nystagmus. Arch Ophthalmol 1979; 97:1877-1885.

Ellenberger C, Netsky MG: Anatomic basis and diagnostic value of opsoclonus. Arch Ophthalmol 1970; 83:307-310.

Gilman N, Baloh RW, Tomiyasu V: Primary position upbeat nystagmus. Neurology 1977; 27:294-298.

Hood ED, Kayan A, Leech J: Rebound nystagmus. Brain 1973; 96:507-526.

Ishikawa S: Latent nystagmus and its etiology. In Reinecke RD (ed): Strabismus: Proceedings of the third meeting of the International Strabismological Association. Kyoto, Japan. New York: Grune & Stratton, 1978, pp. 203-214.

Norton EWD, Cogan DG: Spasmus nutans: a clinical study of 20 cases followed two years or more since onset. Arch Ophthalmol 1954; 52:442-446.

Popper JL, Marino R: Pinealomas and tumors of the posterior portion of the third ventricle. J Neurosurg 1968; 28:357-364.

Schmidt D: Congenital nystagmus. Clinical aspects, In Lennerstrand G, Zee DS, Keller FL (eds): Functional basis of ocular motility disorders. Oxford, Pergamon Press, 1982.

Selhorst JB, Stark L, Ochs AL, et al: Disorders in cerebellar ocular motor control. I. Saccadic over-shoot dysmetria: an oculographic control system and clinico-anatomical analysis. Brain 1976; 99:497-508.

Smith JL, Zieper I, Gay AJ, et al: Nystagmus retractorius. Arch Ophthalmol 1959; 62:864-867.

Susac JO, Hoyt WF, Daroff RB, et al: Clinical spectrum of ocular bobbing. J Neurol Neurosurg Psychiatry 1970; 33:771-775.

Tahmoush AJ, Brooks JE, Keltner JL: Palatal myoclonus associated with abnormal ocular and extremity movements. Arch Neurol 1972; 27:431-440.

Zahn JR: Incidence and characteristics of voluntary nystagmus. J Neurol Neurosurg Psychiatry 1978; 41:617-623.

Zee DS: Mechanisms of nystagmus. Am J Otol (Suppl.) 1985; 6:30-34.

4

The Six Syndromes of the Sixth (Abducens) Nerve

A. Anatomic considerations

1. Figure 4-1 identifies the structures in the posterior fossa, base of the skull, and middle cranial fossa that serve as landmarks in the study of the sixth nerve
2. Figure 4-2 is a schematic representation of these structures and includes a sagittal section of the brainstem
3. Figure 4-3 is a schematic representation of these structures when viewed from the occipital pole
4. Figure 4-4 illustrates the S-shaped course of the sixth nerve and shows its relationship to the seventh and eighth cranial nerves and the internal carotid artery
5. Figure 4-5 adds the third, fourth, and fifth cranial nerves
6. Figure 4-6 shows the composite diagram and the division of the course of the sixth nerve into five portions, each associated with a different syndrome
   VI^1) The brainstem syndrome
   VI^2) Subarachnoid space syndrome
   VI^3) Petrous apex syndrome
   VI^4) The cavernous sinus syndrome
   VI^5) The orbital syndrome

B. The brainstem syndrome (VI^1)

1. Figure 4-6 reminds us that a brainstem lesion of the sixth nerve may also affect V, VII, VIII nerves and the cerebellum
2. Figure 4-7 illustrates the structures within the substance of the lower pons that may be affected by a lesion affecting the sixth nerve
   a. Oculosympathetic central neuron: ipsilateral Horner's syndrome
   b. PPRF: ipsilateral horizontal conjugate gaze palsy
   c. MLF: ipsilateral internuclear ophthalmoplegia
   d. Pyramidal tract: contralateral hemiparesis
3. The brainstem syndrome may consist of any combination of the deficits listed above; the following are frequently encountered syndromes
   a. Millard-Gubler syndrome
      1) Sixth nerve paresis
      2) Ipsilateral seventh nerve paresis
      3) Contralateral hemiparesis

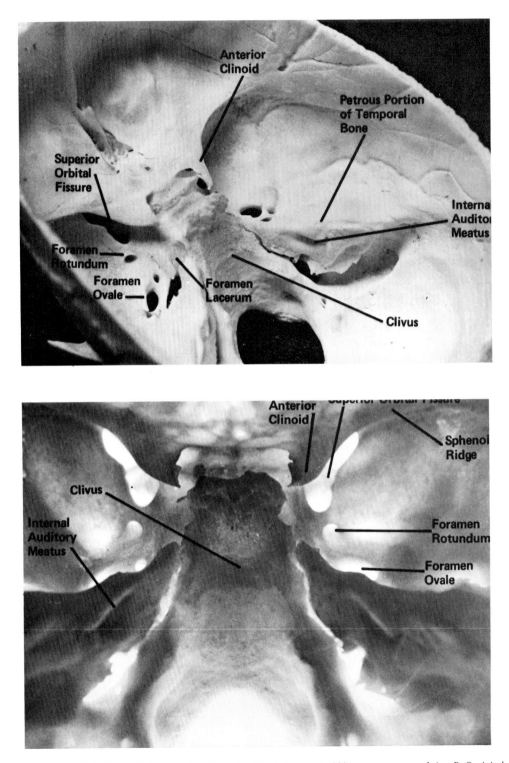

Fig. 4-1. Human skull. Anatomical landmarks in the study of the sixth nerve. A. Oblique superotemporal view. B. Occipital view, retro-illuminated skull.

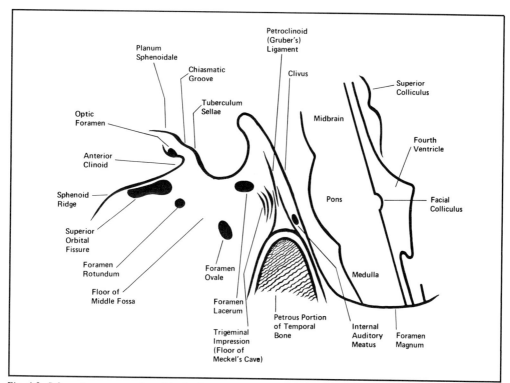

Fig. 4-2. *Schematic representation of the landmarks, temporal view.*

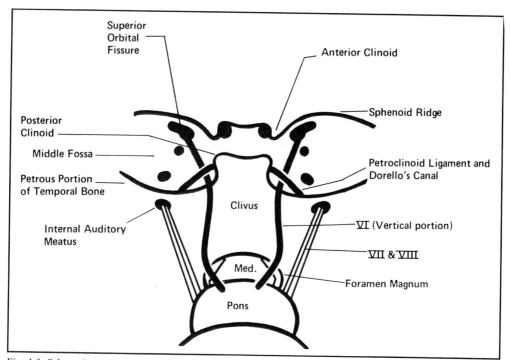

Fig. 4-3. *Schematic representation of the anatomical landmarks, occipital view.*

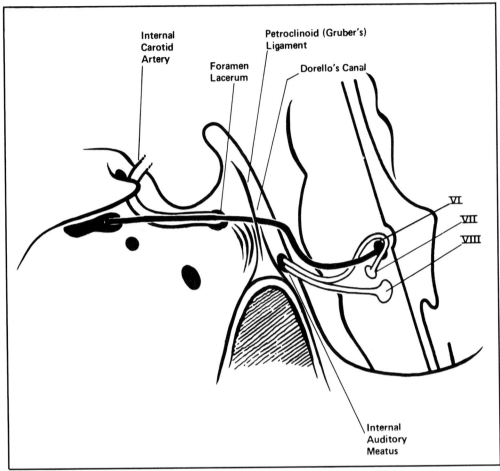

Internal
Carotid
Artery

Foramen
Lacerum

Petroclinoid (Gruber's)
Ligament

Dorello's Canal

VI
VII
VIII

Internal
Auditory
Meatus

Fig. 4-4. Course of the sixth nerve (highlighted in black) from the pons to the superior orbital tissue.

  b. Raymond's syndrome
    1) Sixth nerve paresis
    2) Contralateral hemiparesis
  c. Foville's syndrome
    1) Horizontal conjugate gaze palsy
    2) Ipsilateral V, VII, VIII cranial nerve palsies
    3) Ipsilateral Horner's syndrome

C. The subarachnoid space syndrome (VI²)
  1. Elevated intracranial pressure (ICP) may result in downward displacement of the brainstem, with stretching of the sixth nerve, which is tethered at its exit from the pons and in Dorello's canal
    a. Gives rise to "non-localizing" sixth nerve palsies of raised ICP
    b. Approximately 30% of patients with pseudotumor cerebri have sixth nerve paresis, the only neurologic deficit they are allowed, besides papilledema and its visual field changes

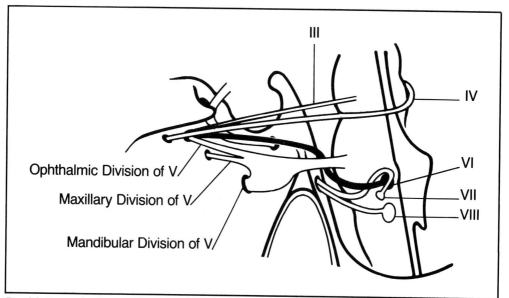

Fig. 4-5. Composite diagram illustrating the third through eighth cranial nerves.

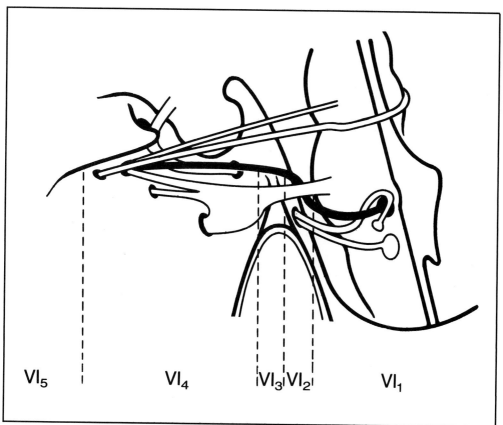

Fig. 4-6. Composite diagram divided into five sections, corresponding to the first five syndromes of the sixth nerve (VI_1-VI_5).

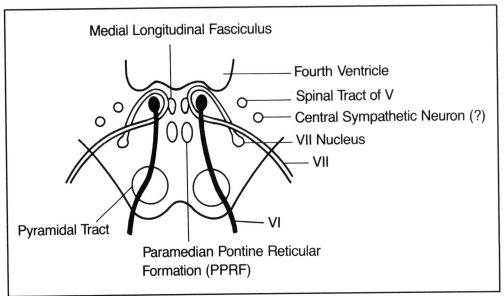

Fig. 4-7. Diagram of cross-section of the lower pons, through the sixth nerve nucleus and fascicle (highlighted in black).

2. Other disturbances in the subarachnoid space causing sixth nerve palsies including hemorrhage, meningeal or parameningeal infection (e.g. viral, bacterial, fungal), inflammation (e.g. sarcoidosis), or infiltration (e.g. lymphoma, leukemia, carcinoma)

D. Petrous apex syndrome (VI[3])

1. Contact with the tip of the petrous pyramid makes the portion of the sixth nerve within Dorello's canal susceptible to pathologic processes affecting the petrous bone
2. Gradenigo's syndrome
   a. Clinical findings
      1) VI nerve palsy
      2) Ipsilateral decreased hearing
      3) Ipsilateral facial pain in the distribution of the V nerve
      4) Ipsilateral facial paralysis
   b. Due to localized inflammation or extradural abscess of petrous apex following complicated otitis media
3. Petrous bone fracture
   a. Basal skull fracture following head trauma
   b. Potential cranial nerve involvement: V, VI, VII, VIII
   c. Associated findings: hemotympanum, Battle's sign, CSF otorrhea
4. Pseudo-Gradenigo's syndrome
   a. Nasopharyngeal carcinoma: may cause serous otitis media due to obstruction of the eustachian tube, and the carcinoma may subsequently invade the cavernous sinus, causing sixth nerve paresis
   b. Cerebellopontine angle tumor: may cause sixth nerve paresis and other

clinical findings, including
1) Decreased hearing
2) VII nerve palsy
3) V nerve paralysis
4) Ataxia
5) Papilledema

E. The cavernous sinus syndrome (VI⁴)

1. Lesions in cavernous sinus rarely produce isolated sixth nerve palsy; associated involvement of
   a. III, IV, Ophthalmic (V¹) nerves
   b. Carotid oculosympathetic plexus (Horner's syndrome)
   c. Optic nerve and chiasm
   d. Pituitary gland
2. Differential diagnosis of cavernous sinus disease includes
   a. Trauma
   b. Vascular
   c. Neoplastic
   d. Inflammatory
3. See Chapter 7

F. The orbital syndrome (VI⁵)

1. Proptosis is an early sign and may be accompanied by congestion of the conjunctival vessels and chemosis
2. The optic nerve may appear normal, or demonstrate atrophy or edema
3. Trigeminal signs are limited to the ophthalmic division
4. It is frequently difficult to distinguish between cranial nerve (III, IV, VI) pareses and mechanical restriction of the globe
5. Etiologies
   a. Tumor (local, metastatic)
   b. Trauma
   c. Inflammatory pseudotumor
   d. Cellulitis

G. Isolated sixth nerve palsy (VI⁶)

1. The sixth syndrome of the sixth nerve
   a. No signs of the first five syndromes
   b. Frequently seen as a post-viral syndrome in young patients and as an ischemic mononeuropathy in adults
   c. As a general rule
      1) Ocular motor cranial nerve palsy in young patient—greater likelihood of neoplasm—aggressive workup
      2) Ocular motor cranial nerve palsy in older patient—greater the likelihood of ischemic mononeuropathy—less aggressive workup
   d. Note in Robertson's series in Table 4-1 (see below) that if cases due to trauma are excluded, a child with a sixth nerve palsy has a 50-50 chance of harboring a neoplasm, usually a brainstem glioma
2. Initial evaluation

TABLE 4-1
ETIOLOGIES OF ACQUIRED VI NERVE PALSY

	Rucker (1958)	Schrader (1960) (Isolated VI)	Rucker (1966)	Johnston (1968)	Robertson (1970) (Children)	Rush (1981)
Total Number of Patients	545	104	607	158	133	419
Etiologies (%)						
Neoplasm	21	7	33	13	39	15
Trauma	16	3	12	32	20	17
Aneurysm	6	0	3	1	3	3
Ischemic	11	36	8	16	0	18
Miscellaneous	16	30	24	30	29	18
Undetermined	30	24	20	8	9	29

    a. Blood pressure determination

    b. Blood tests

        1) CBC

        2) GTT

        3) Sedimentation rate

        4) VDRL and FTA—ABS

        5) ANA (antinuclear antibody)

    c. Radiographic studies

        1) Skull series

        2) Stereoscopic submental-vertex basal view of the skull, for inspection of basal foramina

        3) If the sixth nerve palsy has not shown marked improvement in four months, or if other cranial nerve involvement occurs, then recommend comprehensive evaluation

            a) Medical and neurologic examinations

            b) CT scan with and without contrast

            c) Magnetic resonance imaging (MRI)

            d) Lumbar puncture

            e) Cerebral angiography

H. Table 4-1 contains a summary of six retrospective studies of patients with paresis of the sixth nerve

    1. 8-30%, etiology undetermined, reflecting the vulnerability of the nerve to influences which are transient, benign, and unrecognizable

    2. 16-30% attributed to a miscellaneous group of causes that includes leukemia, migraine, pseudotumor cerebri, multiple sclerosis, myelography; that miscellaneous group of etiologies reflects the poor localizing value of paresis of the sixth nerve

I. The six impostors of the sixth nerve

1. Thyroid eye disease
2. Myasthenia gravis
3. Duane's syndrome (Type I)
4. Spasm of the near reflex
5. Medial wall orbital blow-out fracture with restrictive myopathy
6. Break in fusion of a congenital esophoria

Bibliography

CHAPTERS

Glaser JS: Neuro-ophthalmology, in Duane TD (ed): Clinical Ophthalmology. Hagerstown, Harper & Row, 1978, Vol. 2, Chapter 12.

Miller NR: Walsh and Hoyt's Clinical Neuro-ophthalmology. Baltimore, Williams & Wilkins, 1985, Chapter 35, pp. 652-784.

ARTICLES

Cogan DG: Extraocular muscles and their diseases, in Smith JL (ed): Neuro-ophthalmology. St. Louis, CV Mosby, 1967; Vol. 3, p. 16.

Cogan DG, Freese CG: Spasm of the near reflex. Arch Ophthalmol 1955; 54:753-759.

Cunningham RD: Divergence paralysis. Am J Ophthalmol 1972; 74:630-633.

Duane A: Congenital deficiency of abduction associated with impairment of adduction, retraction movements, contraction of the palpebral fissure, and oblique movements of the eye. Arch Ophthalmol 1905; 34:133-159.

Godtfredsen E, Lederman M: Diagnostic and prognostic roles of ophthalmic neurologic signs and symptoms in malignant nasopharyngeal tumors. Am J Ophthalmol 1965; 59:1063-1069.

Gradenigo G: A special syndrome of endocranial otitic complications (paralysis of the motor oculi externus of otitic origin). Ann Otol 1904; 13:637.

Hotchkiss MG, Miller NR, Clark AW, et al: Bilateral Duane's retraction syndrome. A clinical pathologic case report. Arch Ophthalmol 1980; 98:870-874.

Huber A: Electrophysiology of the retraction syndromes. Br J Ophthalmol 1974; 58:293-300.

Johnston AC: Etiology and treatment of abducens palsy. Trans Pac Coast Oto-ophthalmol Soc 1968; 49:259-277.

Keane JR: Bilateral sixth nerve palsy: analysis of 125 cases. Arch Neurol 1976; 33:681-683.

Knox D, Clark D, Schuster F: Benign VI nerve palsies in children. Pediatrics 1967; 40:560-564.

Moster ML, Savino PJ, Sergott RC, et al: Isolated sixth nerve palsies in younger adults. Arch Ophthalmol 1984; 102:1328-1330.

Robertson DM, Hines JD, Rucker CW: Acquired sixth nerve paresis in children. Arch Ophthalmol 1970; 83:574-579.

Rucker CW: Paralysis of the third, fourth, and sixth cranial nerves. Am J Ophthalmol 1958; 46:787-794.

Rucker CW: The causes of paralysis of the third, fourth, and sixth cranial nerves. Am J Ophthalmol 1966; 61:1293-1298.

Rush JA, Younge BR: Paralysis of cranial nerves III, IV and VI. Cause and prognosis in 1,000 cases. Arch Ophthalmol 1981; 99:76-79.

Sakalas R, Harbison JW, Vines FS, and Becker DP: Chronic sixth nerve palsy. An initial sign of basisphenoid tumors. Arch Ophthalmol 1975; 93:186-190.

Savino PJ, Hilliker JK, Cassell GH, et al: Chronic sixth nerve palsies. Arch Ophthalmol 1982; 100:1442-1444.

Shrader EC, Schlezinger NS: Neuro-ophthalmologic evaluation of abducens nerve paralysis. Arch Ophthalmol 1960; 63:1184-1191.

Smith JL: Pseudotumor cerebrei. Trans Am Acad Ophthalmol Otolaryngol 1958; 62:432-439.

Thomas JE, Yoss RE: The parasellar syndrome: problems of determining etiology. Mayo Clinic Proc 1970; 45:617-623.

Van Meter WS, Younge BR, Harner SG: Ophthalmic manifestations of acoustic neurinoma. Ophthalmology 1983; 90:917-922.

5

The Seven Syndromes of the Third (Oculomotor) Nerve

A. Anatomic considerations

1. Figure 5-1 represents a cross section through the rostral midbrain at the level of the superior colliculi
2. Figure 5-2 is a copy of Figure 5-1 with superimposition of numbers 1 through 6, representing six sites in which the third cranial nerve may be affected and present with distinct ocular manifestations, or in the company of different neurological signs and symptoms, or as a result of specific disease processes. The seventh syndrome is the isolated third nerve palsy
3. Figure 5-3 illustrates the relationship of the third nerve (highlighted in black) to other cranial nerves

B. The seven syndromes of the third nerve

1. Nuclear third nerve paresis (Fig. 5-2, site 1)
   a. Extremely rare
   b. The arrangement of the third nerve subnuclei places strict prerequisites on the diagnosis of a nuclear third nerve palsy
      1) Each superior rectus is innervated by the contralateral third nerve nucleus; therefore, a nuclear third nerve palsy on one side requires paresis of the contralateral superior rectus
      2) Both levators are innervated by one subnuclear structure, the central caudal nucleus; therefore, a nuclear third nerve palsy requires bilateral ptosis
   c. Some cases of skew deviation may actually represent incidences of one or more third nerve subnuclei (subserving the vertical recti or the inferior oblique) being affected
2. Third nerve fascicle syndrome (Fig. 5-2, site 2)
   a. Topical diagnosis depends upon the coexistence of other neurologic signs
   b. Fascicles have already left the third nerve nucleus, so that the ocular manifestations are present only on one side (no longer subject to the rules governing nuclear third nerve paresis)
   c. Nothnagel's syndrome
      1) Lesion in the area of the superior cerebellar peduncle
      2) Ipsilateral third nerve paresis and cerebellar ataxia
   d. Benedikt's syndrome

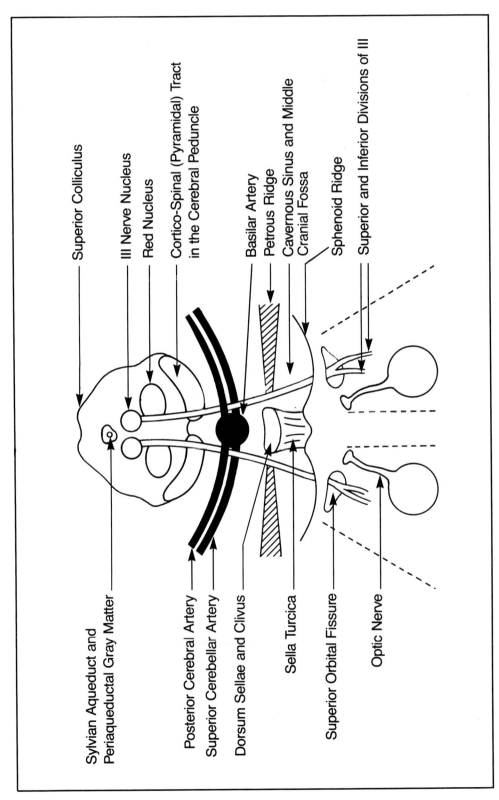

Superior Colliculus

III Nerve Nucleus

Red Nucleus

Cortico-Spinal (Pyramidal) Tract
in the Cerebral Peduncle

Basilar Artery

Petrous Ridge

Cavernous Sinus and Middle
Cranial Fossa

Sphenoid Ridge

Superior and Inferior Divisions of III

Sylvian Aqueduct and
Periaqueductal Gray Matter

Posterior Cerebral Artery

Superior Cerebellar Artery

Dorsum Sellae and Clivus

Sella Turcica

Superior Orbital Fissure

Optic Nerve

Fig. 5-1

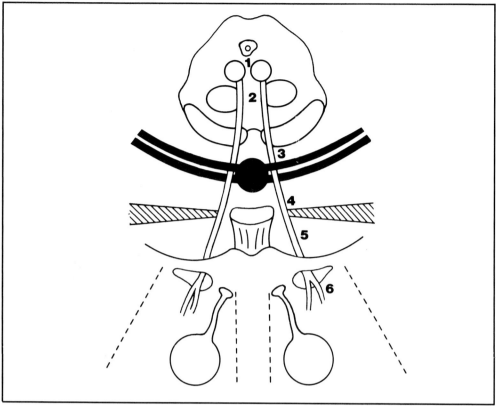

Fig. 5-2

      1) Lesion in the region of the red nucleus
      2) Ipsilateral third nerve paresis with contralateral hemitremor
  e. Weber's syndrome
      1) Involvement of the third nerve in the neighborhood of the cerebral peduncle
      2) Ipsilateral third nerve paresis with contralateral hemiparesis
  f. Claude's syndrome
      1) Features of both Benedikt's and Nothnagel's syndromes
  g. Fascicular lesions are virtually always ischemic, infiltrative (tumor) or, rarely, inflammatory
3. Uncal herniation syndrome (Fig. 5-2, site 3)
  a. In its course toward the cavernous sinus, the third nerve rests on the edge of the tentorium cerebelli
  b. The portion of the brain overlying the third nerve, at the tentorial edge, is the uncal portion of the undersurface of the temporal lobe
  c. A supratentorial space-occupying mass, located anywhere in or above this cerebral hemisphere, may cause a downward displacement and herniation of the uncus across the tentorial edge, thereby compressing the third nerve (Fig. 5-4)

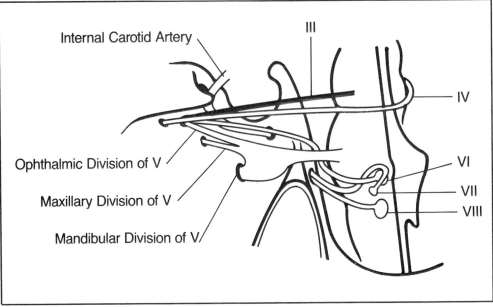

Internal Carotid Artery

III

IV

Ophthalmic Division of V

Maxillary Division of V

Mandibular Division of V

VI

VII

VIII

Fig. 5-3

    d. A dilated and fixed pupil (Hutchinson pupil) may be the first indication that altered consciousness is due to a space-occupying intracranial lesion

4. Posterior communicating artery aneurysm (Fig. 5-2, site 4)
    a. In its course toward the cavernous sinus, the third nerve travels alongside (lateral to) the posterior communicating artery
    b. The most common cause of non-traumatic isolated third nerve paresis with pupillary involvement is an aneurysm at the junction of the posterior communicating artery and the internal carotid artery (Fig. 5-5)
    c. Hemorrhage suddenly enlarges the aneurysmal sac to which the third nerve is adherent or there is actual hemorrhage into the substance of the nerve

5. Cavernous sinus syndrome (Fig. 5-2, site 5)
    a. Third nerve paresis usually seen in association with other cranial nerve involvement: IV, V, VI, oculosympathetic paralysis
    b. Third nerve paresis due to cavernous sinus lesion tends to be partial, i.e. all muscles innervated by the third nerve are not equally involved
    c. Pupillary fibers frequently "spared" such that the pupil may be normal or minimally involved
    d. Cavernous sinus lesions may lead to primary aberrant regeneration of the third nerve (see below)
    e. See Chapter 7

6. Orbital syndrome (Fig. 5-2, site 6)
    a. See the orbital syndrome of the sixth nerve (Chapter 4)
    b. Just before entering the superior orbital fissure, the third nerves split into two divisions

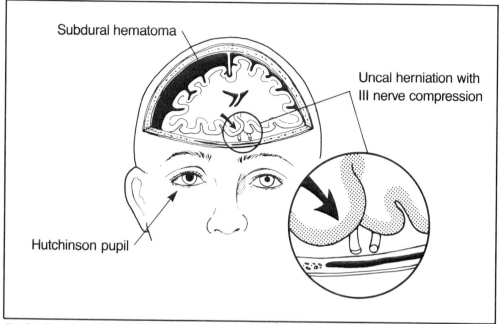

Fig. 5-4. Transtentorial herniation of uncus with third nerve compression.

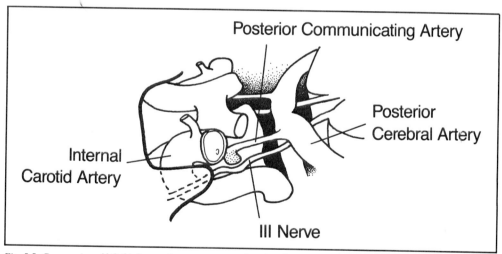

Fig. 5-5. Compression of left third nerve due to aneurysm at junction of posterior communicating and internal carotid arteries.

   c. The superior division innervates the
      1) Superior rectus
      2) Levator palpebrae
   d. The inferior division innervates the
      1) Inferior rectus
      2) Medial rectus
      3) Inferior oblique

TABLE 5-1

ETIOLOGIES OF ACQUIRED III NERVE PALSY

	Rucker (1958)	Goldstein (1960) (Isolated III)	Green (1966)	Rucker (1966)	Rush (1981)
Total Number of Patients	**335**	**61**	**130**	**274**	**290**
Etiologies (%)					
Neoplasm	11	10	4	18	12
Trauma	15	8	11	13	16
Aneurysm	19	18	30	18	14
Ischemic*	19	47	19	17	21
Miscellaneous	8	6	13	12	14
Undetermined	28	11	23	20	23

*Including diabetes mellitus

    4) Pupil (iris sphincter muscle)

    5) Accommodation (ciliary muscle)

  e. Orbital involvement of the third nerve may result in selective paresis of structures innervated by only one of the divisions

7. Pupil-sparing isolated third nerve paresis (the seventh syndrome of the third nerve)

  a. The pupillomotor fibers of the third nerve travel in the outer layers of the nerve and are therefore closer to the nutrient blood supply enveloping the nerve

  b. This may explain why the pupillomotor fibers are spared in 80% of ischemic third nerve pareses, but are affected in 95% of cases of compressive (trauma, tumor, aneurysm) third nerve paresis

  c. Patients with pupil-sparing isolated third nerve palsies are evaluated and managed in a similar manner to patients with isolated fourth and sixth nerve pareses

    1) "Ischemia" lab workup

      a) Blood pressure determination

      b) CBC

      c) Sedimentation rate

      d) Glucose tolerance test

      e) VDRL and FTA—ABS

      f) ANA (antinuclear antibody)

    2) Radiographic studies

      a) Skull series, looking at sella, and sphenoid sinus

          b) Stereoscopic submental-vertex basal view of the skull

      3) If:

          a) The third nerve paresis is truly isolated

          b) And the patient is over 40 years of age

          c) Or has a history of migraine, diabetes, or hypertension
then
Follow the patient for three to four months

      4) Most patients with ischemic third nerve paresis demonstrate improvement of the motility measurements within one month and may have complete recovery by three months (maximum: six months)

      5) If

          a) No significant improvement in three months

          b) Or if the patient develops signs of aberrant regeneration of the third nerve

          c) Or other neurologic findings develop
Then
Recommend cranial CT scanning, MRI scanning, and four-vessel cerebral angiography

      6) CAUTION: ocular myasthenia can mimic a pupil-sparing third nerve palsy; remember the Tensilon test!

C. Incidence of various causes of third nerve palsies

    1. Table 5-1 summarizes five major published series of patients with paresis of the oculomotor nerve

    2. Although neoplasm, aneurysm and ischemia are the most common etiologies, 10% to 25% of cases of third nerve palsies have an undetermined cause

D. Aberrant regeneration (misdirection) of the third nerve

    1. Regeneration of the disrupted third nerve fibers may result in fibers of one structure being hooked up ("axon sprouting") to fibers that terminate in another structure

    2. Clinical phenomena may be classified as

      a. Lid-gaze dyskinesis

         1) Some of the inferior rectus fibers may end up innervating the levator, so that the lid retracts when the patient looks down: pseudo-von Graefe's sign

         2) Some of the medial rectus fibers may end up supplying some of the innervation to the levator, so that the lid retracts when the patient adducts his eye: inverse Duane's syndrome

      b. Pupil-gaze dyskinesis

         1) Some of the medial rectus fibers may end up innervating the pupillary sphincter muscle, so that there is more pupil constriction during convergence than as a response to light: pseudo-Argyll Robertson pupil

         2) Some of the fibers destined to innervate the inferior rectus may end up innervating the pupillary sphincter, so that on attempted downgaze the pupil constricts

3. Two forms of aberrant regeneration
    a. Primary aberrant regeneration
        1) No preceding acute third nerve palsy
        2) Insidious development of third nerve palsy with accompanying signs of misdirection
        3) Sign of an intracavernous lesion: meningioma, aneurysm, neurinoma
    b. Secondary aberrant regeneration
        1) Observe weeks to months during recovery from a third nerve palsy
        2) Seen after trauma and tumor compression of the third nerve, but never after ischemic third nerve paresis. If you are following a patient with a presumed diagnosis of ischemic third nerve palsy, and he develops signs of aberrant regeneration, then CT scanning and cerebral angiography are indicated

E. Rare causes of third nerve paresis

1. Ophthalmoplegic migraine
    a. Onset almost always in childhood
    b. Usually a family history of migraine
    c. Third nerve paresis may occur at any time in relation to headache, but usually appears as the headache phase abates
    d. As a rule, third nerve palsy clears completely within one month, but occasionally permanent oculomotor paresis occurs
2. Cyclic oculomotor palsy
    a. Disorder usually present at birth or early in childhood
    b. Occurs in a setting of a total third nerve palsy
    c. Spastic movements of the muscles innervated by the third nerve results in lid elevation, adduction, miosis, and increased accommodation
    d. These movements occur at regular intervals, lasting 10-30 seconds
    e. Etiology unknown

Bibliography

CHAPTERS

Glaser JS: Neuro-ophthalmology, In Duane TD (ed.): Clinical Ophthalmology. Hagerstown, Harper & Row, 1978, Vol. 2, Chapter 12.

Miller NR: Walsh and Hoyt's Clinical Neuro-ophthalmology. Baltimore, Williams & Wilkins, 1985, Chapter 35, pp. 652 784.

ARTICLES

Asbury AK, Aldredge H, Hirshberg R, et al: Oculomotor palsy in diabetes mellitus: a clinicopathological study. Brain 1970; 93:555-566.

Cox TA, Wurster JB, Godfrey WA: Primary aberrant oculomotor regeneration due to intracranial aneurysm. Arch Neurol 1979; 36:570-571.

Derakhshan I: Superior branch palsy of the oculomotor nerve with spontaneous recovery. Ann Neurol 1978; 4:478-479.

Eyster EF, Hoyt WF, Wilson CB: Oculomotor palsy from minor head trauma. An initial sign of basal intracranial tumor. JAMA 1972; 220:1083-1086.

Friedman AP, Harter DH, Merritt HH: Ophthalmoplegic migraine. Arch Neurol 1962; 7:320-327.

Goldstein JE, Cogan DG: Diabetic ophthalmoplegia with special reference to the pupil. Arch Ophthalmol 1960; 64:592-600.

Green WR, Hackett ER, Schlezinger NS: Neuro-ophthalmologic evaluation of oculomotor nerve paralysis. Arch Ophthalmol 1964; 72:154-167.

Kerr FWL, Hollowell OW: Location of pupillomotor and accommodation fibers in the oculomotor nerve: Experimental observation in paralytic mydriasis. J Neurol Neurosurg Psychiatry 1964; 27:473-481.

Kissel JT, Burde RM, Klingele TG, et al: Pupil-sparing oculomotor palsies with internal carotid-posterior communicating artery aneurysms. Ann Neurol 1983; 13:149-154.

Loewenfeld IE, Thompson HS: Oculomotor paresis with cyclic spasms. A critical review of the literature and a new case. Surv Ophthalmol 1975; 20:81-124.

Rucker CW: Paralysis of the third, fourth, and sixth cranial nerves. Am J Ophthalmol 1958; 46:787-794.

Rucker CW: The causes of aralysis of the third, fourth, and sixth cranial nerves. Am J Ophthalmol 1966; 61:1293-1298.

Rush JA, Younge BR: Paralysis of careful nerves III, IV, and VI. Cause and prognosis in 1,000 cases. Arch Ophthalmol 1981; 99:76-79.

Schatz NJ, Savino PJ, Corbett JJ: Primary aberrant oculomotor regeneration. A sign of intracavernous meningioma. Arch Neurol 1977; 34:29-32.

Soni SR: Aneurysms of the posterior communicating artery and oculomotor paresis. J Neurol Neurosurg Psychiatry 1974; 37:475-484.

Susac JO, Hoyt WF: Inferior branch palsy of the oculomotor nerve. An Neurol 1977; 2:336-339.

Walsh FB: Third nerve regeneration: A clinical evaluation. Br J Ophthalmol 1957; 41:577-598.

Warwick R: Representation of the extraocular muscles in the oculomotor nuclei of the markey. J Comp Neurol 1953; 98:449-495.

Weber RB, Daroff RB, Mackey EA: Pathology of oculomotor nerve palsy in diabetics. Neurology 1970; 20:835-838.

6

Five Syndromes of the Fourth (Trochlear) Nerve

A. Anatomic Considerations

1. Figure 6-1 is a diagram of a cross section of the lower midbrain at the level of the inferior colliculi
2. The fourth nerve is
   a. The only cranial nerve that exits at the dorsal aspect of the brainstem (Fig. 6-2)
   b. The cranial nerve with the longest intracranial course (75 mm)
3. The fourth nerve fascicles cross in the anterior medullary velum (anterior floor of the fourth ventricle) prior to exiting dorsally and coursing anteriorly around the midbrain to travel forward between the superior cerebellar and posterior cerebral arteries (just as, but laterally separated from, the third cranial nerve)
4. Therefore, the left fourth nerve fascicle become the right fourth nerve and innervates the right superior oblique muscle; and the right fourth nerve fascicle becomes the left fourth nerve and innervates the left superior oblique muscle

B. Clinical syndromes of the fourth nerve (Fig. 6-3)—Nuclear-fascicular syndrome, Subarachnoid space syndrome, Cavernous sinus syndrome, Orbital syndrome, Isolated fourth nerve palsy (Congenital or Acquired)

1. Nuclear-fascicular syndrome (Fig. 6-3, site 1)
   a. Distinguishing nuclear from fascicular lesions is virtually impossible due to the short course of the fascicles within the midbrain, and thus the lack of associated neurologic signs
   b. Frequent etiologies include hemorrhage, infarction, demyelination, trauma (including neurosurgical)
   c. Fascicular lesion may be seen with contralateral Horner's syndrome, since the sympathetic pathways descend through the dorsolateral tegmentum of the midbrain adjacent to the trochlear fascicles
2. Subarachnoid space syndrome (Fig. 6-3, site 2)
   a. Fourth nerve particularly susceptible to injury as it emerges from dorsal surface of brainstem
   b. When bilateral fourth nerve palsies occur, the site of injury is likely in the anterior medullary velum. Contracoup forces transmitted to the brainstem

97

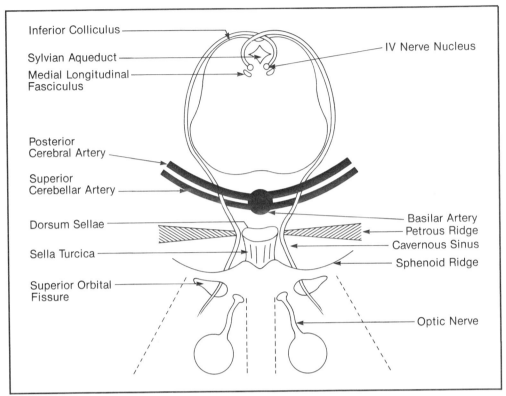

Inferior Colliculus

Sylvian Aqueduct

Medial Longitudinal
Fasciculus

IV Nerve Nucleus

Posterior
Cerebral Artery

Superior
Cerebellar Artery

Dorsum Sellae

Sella Turcica

Superior Orbital
Fissure

Basilar Artery
Petrous Ridge
Cavernous Sinus
Sphenoid Ridge

Optic Nerve

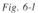

Fig. 6-1

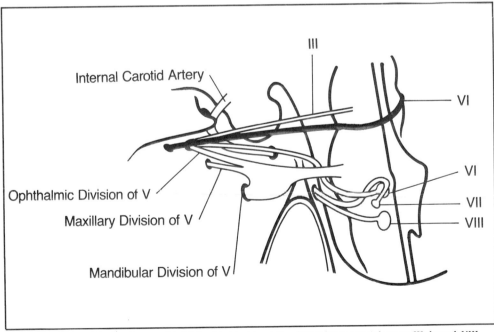

III

Internal Carotid Artery

VI

VI

Ophthalmic Division of V

Maxillary Division of V

VII

VIII

Mandibular Division of V

Fig. 6-2. Diagram of the fourth nerve (highlighted in black) and its relationship to cranial nerves III through VIII.

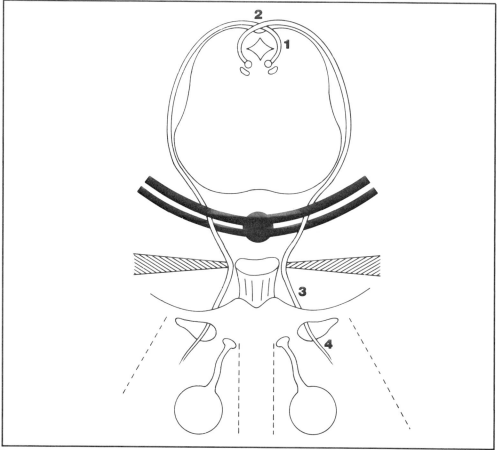

Fig. 6-3

    by the free tentorial edge may injure the nerves at this site
  c. Less frequent causes include tumor (e.g. pinealoma, tentorial meningioma), meningitis, neurosurgical trauma
3. Cavernous sinus syndrome (Fig. 6-3, site 3)
  a. Seen in association with other cranial nerve palsies: III, V, VI oculosympathetic paralysis
  b. Checking fourth nerve function in the setting of a third nerve paresis
    1) Since the involved eye cannot be adducted well, the vertical actions of the superior oblique muscle cannot be tested
    2) Therefore, the eye is moved into abduction and then the patient is instructed to look down; the ability of the eye to intort is examined, as a measure of fourth nerve function
    3) If a limbal or conjunctival landmark (e.g. pterygium or blood vessel) is noted to intort, then the fourth nerve is presumed intact
  c. See Chapter 7
4. Orbital syndrome (Fig. 6-3, site 4)

99

Parks-Bielschowsky 3-Step Test

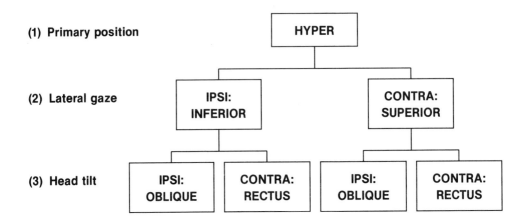

(1) Primary position

(2) Lateral gaze

(3) Head tilt

ALWAYS THINK IN TERMS OF <u>PARETIC</u> MUSCLE

Courtesy of F.J. Elsas, M.D.

Fig. 6-4

    a. Usually seen in association with other cranial nerve palsies: III, V, VI; and orbital signs including proptosis, chemosis, conjunctival injection

    b. Major etiologies include trauma, inflammation, tumor

  5. Isolated fourth nerve palsy

    a. Congenital

      1) See below (section F) for incidence of this condition

      2) Most often seen in pediatric population and late in life (5th to 7th decades) as patient's fourth nerve palsy may decompensate

      3) Diagnostic keys

        a) Large vertical fusion amplitude (10-15 prism diopters)

        b) F.A.T. scan (family album tomography): look at old photographs to detect longstanding head tilt, indicative of congenital etiology

    b. Acquired

      1) Acute onset of vertical diplopia, usually with torsional component

      2) Characteristic head position

        a) Tilt to opposite shoulder

        b) Head turn downward with chin depressed, eyes up

        c) Face turn to opposite side

       3) Must perform Parks-Bielschowsky three-step test (see below) to confirm diagnosis

       4) Initial evaluation

         a) Blood pressure determination

         b) Glucose tolerance test

         c) Sedimentation rate

       5) As with other isolated ocular motor neuropathies, if the fourth nerve palsy has not improved or resolved within four months, or if other neurologic signs develop, further workup is indicated

         a) Medical and neurologic examinations

         b) CT scanning

         c) MRI scanning

         d) Lumbar puncture

         e) Cerebral angiography

C. Diagnosis of recently acquired fourth nerve palsy

1. If a patient has vertical misalignment (hypertropia) due to recently acquired weakness of a single vertically-acting muscle, then we determine the weak muscle by performing the Parks-Bielschowsky 3-step test (Fig. 6-4)

   a. The medial and lateral rectus muscle do not have vertical action

   b. Therefore, hypertropia (HT) of paretic etiology is caused by weakness of one or more of the following eight vertically-acting muscles

      Right inferior oblique (RIO); left inferior oblique (LIO)

      Right superior oblique (RSO); left superior oblique (LSO)

      Right inferior rectus (RIR); left inferior rectus (LIR)

      Right superior rectus (RSR); left superior rectus (LSR)

   c. If the HT is due to weakness of only one of these eight muscles, the paretic muscle is identified by answering the three questions asked in the Parks-Bielschowsky 3-step test

   d. Each step cuts the possible number of muscles in half

      1) After the first step, there are four possible muscles remaining

      2) After the second step, there are two remaining

      3) After the third step, only the one guilty muscle remains

   e. Parks-Bielschowsky first-step: which is the higher eye?

      1) If the patient has an RHT then the weak muscle is either a depressor of the right eye (RIR, RSO) or an elevator of the left eye (LSR, LIO)

      2) If the patient has a LHT then the weak muscle is either an elevator of the right eye (RSR, RIO) or a depressor of the left eye (LIR, LSO)

      3) Therefore, by determining if the patient has an RHT or an LHT, you have narrowed down the number of suspected muscles from 8 to 4

   f. Parks-Bielschowsky second-step: HT worse on gaze right or left?

      1) The vertical rectus muscles (superior and inferior recti) have their greatest vertical action (and least torsional action) when the eye is abducted

      2) Therefore, LHT due to paresis of LIR will be worse on gaze left (since OS is abducted on gaze left); LHT due to paresis of RSR will be worse

on gaze right (since OD is abducted on right gaze)

3) The oblique muscles (superior and inferior obliques) have their greatest vertical action (at least torsional action) when the eye is adducted

4) Therefore, LHT due to paresis of LSO will be worse on gaze right; LHT due to paresis of RIO, will be worse on gaze left

5) LHT worse on gaze right is due to weakness of either LSO or RSR

6) LHT worse on gaze left is due to weakness of either LIR or RIO

7) Thus, in the case of LHT, by answering the question: "LHT worse on gaze right or left?" You have narrowed the possible muscles from four (LSO, RSR, LIR, RIO) to two (either LSO-RS, or LIR-RIO)

8) Similarly, the possible causes of RHT is narrowed down from four (RIR, LIO, LSR, RSO) to two (RIR-LIO if RHT worse on gaze right; LSR-RIO if RHT worse on gaze left)

9) Note: In each case
   a) RHT worse on gaze right (RIR or LIO)
   b) RHT worse on gaze left (RSO or LSR)
   c) LHT worse on gaze right (LSO or RSR)
   d) LHT worse on gaze left (RIO or LIR)
      You are left with either two superior or two inferior muscles; and "one will be a rectus and one an oblique" and "one will be of the right eye and one of the left." If this is not the case (e.g. if you have narrowed it down, after the second step, to "RIR vs. LSR" or "LSO vs. LIO") then you have made a mistake and need to retrace your steps!

g. Parks-Bielschowsky third-step: Is the HT worse on head-tilt right (head tilted so that the right ear is near the right shoulder) or head-tilt left (head tilted so that the left ear is near the left shoulder)?

   1) The superior muscles (SR and SO) intort the eyes; the inferior muscles (IR and IO) extort the eye

   2) When the head is tilted downward to the right shoulder the eyes undergo corrective torsion (i.e., OD intorted and OS extorted)

   3) Therefore, when the head is tilted to the right, OD will be intorted by contraction of RSR and RSO; these two muscles work together in effecting the intorsion, and neutralize each other's vertical action (RSR is an elevator and RSO a depressor)

   4) If one of these muscles is the paretic muscle responsible for the HT, then the vertical action will not be neutralized and the HT will be worse on tilting the head to the right shoulder

   5) Therefore, the mnemonic for the third step is
      a) If you are left with two superior muscles then the paretic muscle is the one on the same side as the shoulder toward which the head-tilt makes the HT worse; e.g., if it is narrowed down to "RSO vs. LSR" then the paretic muscle is "RSO if RHT worse on tilt to right" and "LSR if RHT is worse to tilt left"
      b) If you are left with two inferior muscles, then the paretic muscle is

TABLE 6-1
ETIOLOGIES OF ACQUIRED IV NERVE PALSY

	Rucker (1958)	Rucker (1966)	Khawam (1967)	Burger (1970)	Younge (1977)	Rush (1981)
Total Number of Patients	**67**	**84**	**40**	**33**	**36**	**172**
Etiologies (%)						
Neoplasm	4	8	2.5	21	0	4
Trauma	36	27	67.5	39	44	32
Aneurysm	0	0	0	3	0	2
Ischemic	36	15	2.5	18	33	18
Miscellaneous	10	15	7.5	9	8	4
Undetermined	13	33	20	6	15	36

the one on the side opposite the shoulder toward which the head-tilt makes the HT worse; e.g., if it is narrowed down to "RIO vs. LIR" then the paretic muscle is "RIO if LHT worse on tilt left" and "LIR if LHT worse on tilt right"

2. Bajandas described Bielschowsky's "missing step": Is the HT worse on gaze up or gaze down?
    a. This step confirms step 3
    b. Note again, that after step 2, we are down to either two superior or two inferior muscles
        1) RSR vs. LSO
        2) RSO vs. LSR
        3) RIR vs. LIO
        4) RIO vs. LIR
3. Note also that in each case, one muscle is an elevator and the other a depressor
4. Therefore, we can confirm the paretic muscle identified by step 3 by noting if the HT is worse on gaze up (RSR, LSR, LIO, RIO) or gaze down (LSO, RSO, RIR, LIR)

D. Measuring torsional component of fourth nerve palsy
    1. Double Maddox rod test to quantitate torsional component of diplopia
    2. The patient will report intorsion of image seen by eye with fourth nerve palsy. Actually, this indicates excyclotorsion of the patient's eye, caused by overaction of the antagonist inferior oblique muscle
    3. Greater than 10° of torsion is suggestive of bilateral fourth nerve palsies

E. Bilateral fourth nerve palsies
    1. Usually due to severe head trauma, with contusion of the anterior medullary velum where the fourth nerve fascicles cross

    2. Parks-Bielschowsky 3-step test

      a. Either eye may be hypertropic in primary position, or patient may be orthophoric

      b. RHT on gaze left; LHT on gaze right

      c. RHT on head-tilt right; LHT on head-tilt left

    3. With double Maddox rods, measure greater than 10° of torsion

F. Incidence of various causes of fourth nerve palsy

    1. Table 6-1 summarizes six large series of patients with acquired paresis of the fourth nerve

    2. Summary of cases of acquired, isolated fourth paresis (10-20-30-40 rule)

      a. 10%: neoplasm-aneurysm

      b. 20%: ischemic

      c. 30%: undetermined or miscellaneous

      d. 40%: trauma

    3. A large proportion of fourth nerve palsies are classified as congenital. In Harley's series of 18 children, 67% (12/18) were congenital, while in Younge's report of 52 adults, 29% (15/52) were congenital

    4. The frequency of congenital fourth nerve paresis cannot be overemphasized. Many adults presenting in the fifth and sixth decades of life may have decompenated, congenital fourth nerve palsies

G. Differential diagnosis of vertical diplopia

    1. Ocular myasthenia

    2. Thyroid eye disease

    3. Orbital disease (tumor, trauma, inflammation, blow-out fracture of the floor)

    4. Third nerve paresis

    5. Brown's syndrome

    6. Skew deviation

H. Other syndromes of the superior oblique muscle

    1. Brown's (sheath) syndrome

      a. Limitation of elevation of the eye in adduction because movements of the superior oblique tendon in the trochlea are restricted

      b. Affected eye usually hypotropic, and the patient often develops abnormal head position (chin up)

      c. Forced ductions must be positive to establish diagnosis

      d. Congenital etiology: superior oblique tendon is short and tethered

      e. Acquired etiologies

        1) Tenosynovitis may prevent tendon from passing through the trochlear pully

        2) Orbital trauma to trochlear region

    2. Superior oblique myokymia

      a. Unexplained condition causing vertical diplopia or monocular blurred vision with tremulous sensations of the affected eye

      b. Paroxysmal, rapid, vertical and torsional movements of one eye that are usually small, necessitating slit-lamp examination or ophthalmoscopy

c. Precipitated by asking the patient to first look in the direction of action of the superior oblique muscle and then return to the primary position
d. Usually benign; occasionally seen with multiple sclerosis
e. Treatment
 1) Carbamazepine (Tegretol)
 2) Superior oblique surgery

Bibliography

CHAPTERS

Glaser JS: Neuro-ophthalmology, In Duane TD (ed.): Clinical Ophthalmology. Hagerstown, Harper & Row, 1978, Vol. 2, Chapter 12.

Miller NR: Walsh and Hoyt's Clinical Neuro-ophthalmology. Baltimore, Williams & Wilkins, 1985, Chapter 35, pp. 652-784.

ARTICLES

Brown HW: True and simulated superior oblique tendon sheath syndromes. Doc Ophthalmol 1973; 34:123-136.

Burger LJ, Kalvin NH, Smith JL: Acquired lesions of the fourth cranial nerve. Brain 1970; 93:567-574.

Coppeto JR: Superior oblique paresis and contralateral Horner's syndrome. Ann Ophthalmol 1983; 15:681-683.

Harley RD: Paralytic strabismus in children: Etiologic incidence and management of the third, fourth, and sixth nerve palsies. Ophthalmology 1980; 86:24-43.

Hoyt WF, Keane JR: Superior oblique myokymia: report and discussion on five cases of benign intermittent uniocular microtremor. Arch Ophthalmol 1970; 84:461-467.

Khawam E, Scott AB, Jampolsky A: Acquired superior oblique palsy. Arch Ophthalmol 1967; 77:761-768.

Parks MM: Isolated cyclovertical muscle palsy. Arch Ophthalmol 1958; 60:1027-1035.

Rucker CW: Paralysis of the third, fourth, and sixth cranial nerves. Am J Ophthalmol 1958; 46:787-794.

Rucker CW: The causes of paralysis of the third, fourth, and sixth cranial nerves. Am J Ophthalmol 1966; 61:1293-1298.

Rush JA, Younge BR: Paralysis of cranial nerves III, IV, and VI. Cause and prognosis in 1,000 cases. Arch Ophthalmol 1981; 99:76-79.

Susac JO, Smith JL, Schatz NJ: Superior oblique myokymia. Arch Neurol 1973; 29:432-434.

Younge BR, Sutula F: Analysis of trochlear nerve palsies: diagnosis, etiology, and treatment. Mayo Clinic Proc 1977; 52:11-18.

Cavernous Sinus Syndrome

A. General considerations

1. The ocular motor cranial nerves lie in proximity within the cavernous sinus and superior orbital fissure
2. Since the cavernous sinus contains structures that continue through the superior orbital fissure, it is often impossible to state whether a lesion is in the sinus or in the fissure. More general designation is parasellar syndrome
3. Typically, patients present with periorbital or hemicranial pain, combined with ipsilateral ocular motor nerve palsies, oculosympathetic paralysis, and sensory loss in the distribution of the ophthalmic (V^1) and occasionally maxillary (V^2) division of the trigeminal nerve. Clinically, various combinations of these cranial nerve palsies occur
4. The "orbital apex syndrome" should be reserved for multiple ocular motor cranial nerve palsies plus optic nerve dysfunction

B. Anatomy (Figs. 7-1 and 7-2)

1. Traditionally, the cavernous sinus was thought to be an unbroken, trabeculated

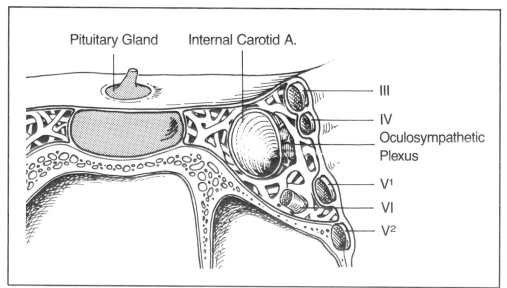

Fig. 7-1. Coronal view of left cavernous and its contents.

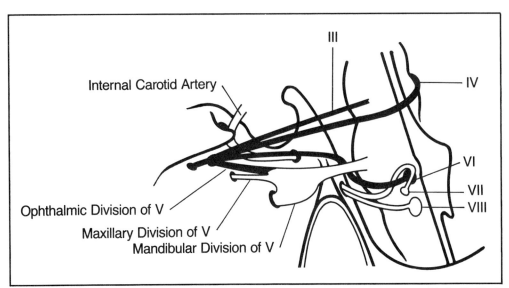

Fig. 7-2. Lateral schematic view of left cavernous sinus with cranial nerves that traverse the sinus highlighted in black.

structure but recent studies demonstrate that it is a plexus of various sized veins that divide and coalesce
  2. Major constituents
     a. Third nerve
     b. Fourth nerve
     c. Sixth nerve
     d. Ophthalmic nerve (V^1)
     e. Sympathetic carotid plexus
     f. Intracavernous carotid artery
  3. The III, IV, V^1, nerves all lie in a lateral wall of the cavernous sinus. The sixth nerve lies freely within the sinus, just lateral to the intracavernous carotid

C. Causes of cavernous sinus syndrome producing painful ophthalmoplegia
  1. Trauma
  2. Vascular
     Intracavernous carotid artery aneurysm
     Posterior cerebral artery aneurysm
     Carotid-cavernous fistula
     Carotid-cavernous thrombosis
  3. Neoplasm
     Primary intracranial tumor
        Pituitary adenoma
        Meningioma
        Craniopharyngioma
        Sarcoma
        Neurofibroma

          Gasserian ganglion
          Neuroma
          Epidermoid
       Primary cranial tumor
          Chordoma
          Chondroma
          Giant-cell tumor
       Local metastases
          Nasopharyngeal tumor
          Cylindroma
          Adamantinoma
          Squamous cell carcinoma
       Distant metastases
          Lymphoma
          Multiple myeloma
          Carcinomatous metastases
   4. Inflammation
      Bacterial: sinusitis; mucocele; periostitis
      Viral: herpes zoster
      Fungal: mucormycosis
      Spirochetal: *Treponema pallidum*
      Mycobacterial: *Mycobacterium tuberculosis*
      Unknown cause: sarcoidosis; Wegener's granulomatosis, Tolosa-Hunt syndrome

D. Of the more common causes of cavernous sinus syndrome, these points deserve emphasis
   1. Intracavernous carotid artery aneurysm
      a. typically produces slowly progressive, unilateral ophthalmoplegia
      b. may become painful
      c. rarely rupture, but this occurrence produces a carotid-cavernous fistula
   2. Carotid-cavernous fistula
      a. due to direct communication between intracavernous carotid and cavernous sinus
      b. high-flow, high-pressure fistula
      c. most common cause is head trauma
      d. clinical picture: chemosis, proptosis, ocular motor nerve palsies, bruit, retinopathy, increased intraocular pressure
   3. Dural-cavernous fistula
      a. due to communication of dural branches of internal or external carotid arteries and cavernous sinus or vessels in region of sinus
      b. low-flow, low-pressure fistula
      c. most commonly occur spontaneously
      d. more subtle clinical picture: don't be fooled into treating these patients for "red eye"

    4. Nasopharyngeal carcinoma
       a. 2-3 times more common in males
       b. Predilection for oriental patients
       c. Varied clinical presentation
          1) Nasal obstruction
          2) Rhinorrhea
          3) Epistaxis
          4) Otitis media
          5) Proptosis
          6) Ipsilateral dry eye
       d. Ninety-five percent of patients with nasopharyngeal carcinoma have sixth nerve paresis at some time during clinical course
       e. Radiologic study of choice: high resolution CT of subcranial soft tissue in region of nasopharynx
       f. Indirect pharyngoscopy and biopsies of the nasopharynx if clinical suspicion high
    5. Two aspects of neoplastic involvement of the parasellar region require particular attention
       a. Mode of onset and clinical course do not prognosticate the type of lesion, i.e. neoplastic disease may have an acute clinical presentation as well as an expected insidious course
       b. High-dose corticosteroid therapy may initially improve signs and symptoms due to neoplasm
    6. Tolosa-Hunt syndrome
       a. Painful ophthalmoplegia due to granulomatous inflammation occurring in the cavernous sinus
       b. Spontaneous remissions may occur after days or weeks
       c. Recurring attacks may occur at intervals of months or years
       d. Systemic steroids usually lead to marked improvement of signs and symptoms within 48 hours
       e. Categorically, diagnosis of exclusion, and patients with this diagnosis require careful follow-up

E. Imitators of cavernous sinus syndrome
    1. Myasthenia
    2. Ocular dysthyroidism
    3. Orbital disease: inflammation, infection, neoplasm, trauma
    4. Diabetic ophthalmoplegia
       a. Typically acute, often painful, mononeuropathy with full recovery within four months
       b. Less frequent occurrence of simultaneous paralysis of multiple ocular motor nerves. Often painful, recurrent and not responsive to steroid therapy
    5. Giant cell arteritis
       a. Single or multiple ocular motor nerve palsies
       b. Produces ischemic necrosis of extraocular muscles

6. Botulism
   a. Occurs in three forms: food-borne, wound, infantile
   b. Ophthalmologic findings include dilated, poorly-reactive pupils, ptosis, and ophthalmoplegia
   c. Affected individuals have nausea, vomiting, associated with facial, pharyngeal and generalized proximal weakness, and no sensory deficits
   d. Botulinum toxin is the most potent poison known, causing cholinergic blockade with only minute quantities
7. Fisher syndrome
   a. Bulbar variant of Guillain-Barré syndrome, characterized by triad of ataxia, arreflexia, ophthalmoplegia
   b. In evolution, this cranial polyneuropathy may mimic unilateral or bilateral ocular motor nerve palsies, but usually progresses to a virtually total ophthalmoplegia with involvement of pupils and accommodation
   c. Patients may also have facial diplegia, respiratory and swallowing difficulties
   c. Often follows a febrile or "viral" illness
   e. Diagnosis confirmed by finding "albumino-cytologic" dissociation on examination of CSF, i.e. elevated protein in the absence of a pleocytosis

Bibliography

ARTICLES

Barricks ME, Traviesa DB, Glaser JS, et al: Ophthalmoplegia in giant cell arteritis. Brain 1977; 100:209-221.

Fisher CM: An unusual variant of acute idiopathic polyneuritis (syndrome of ophthalmoplegia, ataxia, arreflexia). N Engl J Med 1956; 255:57-65.

Harris FS, Rhoton AL: Anatomy of the cavernous sinus. A microsurgical study. J Neurosurg 1976; 45:169-180.

Hasso AN, Pop PM, Thompson JR, et al: High resolution thin section computed tomography of the cavernous sinus. Radio Graphics 1982; 2:83-100.

Hedges TR III, Jones A, Stark L, et al: Botulin ophthalmoplegia: clinical and oculographic observation. Arch Ophthalmol 1983; 101:211-213.

Hunt WE, Meagher JN, LeFever HE, et al: Painful ophthalmoplegia: its relation to indolent inflammation of the cavernous sinus. Neurology 1961; 11:56-62.

Kline LB, Acker JD, Post MJD: Computed tomographic evaluation of the cavernous sinus. Ophthalmology 1982; 89:374-385.

Kline LB: The Tolosa-Hunt Syndrome. Surv Ophthalmol 1982; 27:79-95.

Madsen PH: Carotid-cavernous fistula. Acta Ophthalmol 1970; 48:731-751.

Meadows SP: Intracavernous aneurysm of the internal carotid artery in the cavernous sinus. Arch Ophthalmol 1959; 62:566-574.

Newton TH, Hoyt WF: Dural arteriovenous shunts in the region of the cavernous sinus. Neuroradiology 1970; 1:71-81.

Parkinson D: Anatomy of the cavernous sinus, in Smith JL (ed): Neuro-ophthalmology. St. Louis, CV Mosby, 1972; Vol. 6, pp. 73-101.

Sanders MD, Hoyt WF: Hypoxic ocular sequelae of carotid-cavernous fistulae. Br J Ophthalmol 1969; 53:82-97.

Schatz NJ, Farmer P: Tolosa-Hunt syndrome: the pathology of painful ophthalmoplegia, in Smith JL (ed): Neuro-ophthalmology. St. Louis, CV Mosby, 1972, Vol. 6, pp. 102-112.

Smith JL, Taxdal DSR: Painful ophthalmoplegia: The Tolosa-Hunt syndrome. Am J Ophthalmol 1966; 61:1466-1472.

Smith JL, Wheliss JA: Ocular manifestations of nasopharyngeal tumors. Trans Am Acad Ophthalmol Otolaryngol 1962; 66:659-664.

Thomas JE, Yoss RE: The parasellar syndrome: problems in determining etiology. Mayo Clin Proc 1970; 45:617-623.

Tolosa E: Periarteritic lesions of the carotid siphon with the clinical features of a carotid infraclinoid aneurysm. J Neurol Neurosurg Psychiatry 1954; 17:300-302.

Trobe JD, Glaser JS, Post MJD: Meningiomas and aneurysms of the cavernous sinus. Arch Ophthalmol 1978; 96:457-467.

A. Anatomic considerations
1. Sphincter muscle of the iris
   a. Innervated by parasympathetic fibers originating in the Edinger-Westphal (EW) nucleus, which forms part of the oculomotor nuclear complex in the midbrain
   b. Input that excites the EW nucleus
      1) Light reflex (see Fig. 8-1)
         a) Afferent neurons from retinal ganglion cells to the pretectal area; intercalated neurons from the pretectal complex to EW nuclei; parasympathetic outflow with the oculomotor nerve to the ciliary ganglion, and then to the iris sphincter muscle
         b) Monocular light information is carried by the optic nerve to the chiasm, where half the fibers decussate to the contralateral optic tract, and half the fibers continue in the ipsilateral optic tract
         c) Approximately two-thirds of the way along the optic tract some of the axons leave the tract, enter the brachium of the superior col-

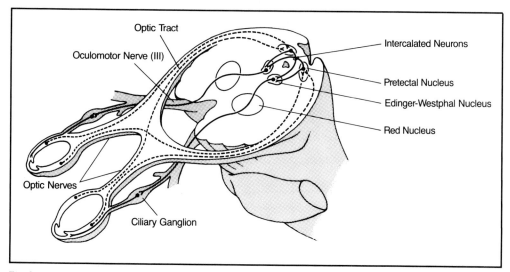

Fig. 8-1. Pathway of the pupillary light reflex (Redrawn from Miller NR: Walsh and Hoyt's Clinical Neuro-ophthalmology. Baltimore, Williams & Wilkins, 1985, p. 421).

liculus, and synapse in the pretectal region

d) The information is then passed forward via the intercalated neurons to the EW nuclei bilaterally

e) The pupillomotor information travels with the third nerve, and beyond the superior orbital fissure, with the inferior division

f) Thus, light information given to one eye is transmitted to both pupils equally

2) Near synkinesis (see Fig. 8-2)

a) The peristriate cortex (area 19), at the upper end of the calcarine fissure, may be the origin of near synkinesis

b) Near synkinesis triad

1. Convergence of eyes

2. Accommodation of the lenses

3. Miosis of the pupils

c) The near synkinesis pathway is more ventrally located than the pretectal afferent limb of the light reflex. This separation of the "near" from "light" reflexes may be the anatomical basis for some instances of light-near dissociation of the pupils (e.g. Argyll Robertson pupils, dorsal midbrain syndrome)

d) The final pathway is the oculomotor nerve, ciliary ganglion, and the short posterior ciliary nerves. The ratio of ciliary ganglion cells

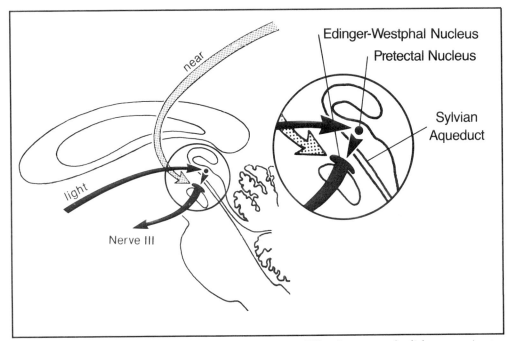

Fig. 8-2. Illustration of more ventral course of near response input to EW nucleus compared to light response input.

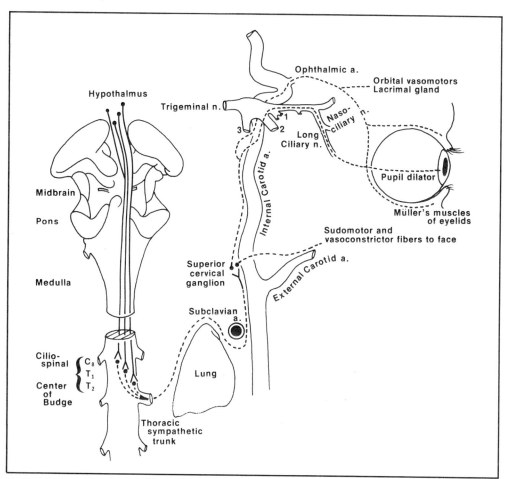

Fig. 8-3. Diagram of oculosympathetic pathway (Reproduced with permission from Glaser J: The Pupils and Accommodation, in Duane TD: Clinical Ophthalmology. Hagerstown, Harper & Row, 1978. Vol. 2, Chap. 15).

which innervate the ciliary muscle vs. cells related to iris sphincter is approximately 30:1

  c. Input that inhibits EW nucleus
    1) Cortical: dilated pupils during epileptic seizures
    2) Spinal-reticular: states of arousal, excitement
    3) Sleep, coma: inhibitory influences decline and pupils are miotic
2. Dilator muscle of the iris
  a. Innervated by sympathetic fibers
  b. Three neuron pathway (see Fig. 8-3)
    1) First-order neuron originates in posterior hypothalamus and courses down through the brainstem to the C8-T2 level of the cord (cilio-spinal center of Budge)
    2) Second-order (preganglionic) neurons leave the cord, enter the para-

vertebral sympathetic chain and terminate in the superior cervical ganglion at the base of the skull

3) Third-order (postganglionic) neuron fibers intended for the pupil and Muller's muscle ascend the internal carotid artery to enter the skull, join the ophthalmic nerve in the cavernous sinus, and then to the orbit through the superior orbital fissure; the sudomotor and vasomotor fibers to the face travel with the external carotid artery

B. Normal pupillary phenomena

1. Physiologic Anisocoria
   a. Approximately 20% of the general population have clearly perceptible anisocoria. The degree of anisocoria can vary from day to day and even switch sides
2. Pupillary unrest
   a. During distance fixation and with constant, moderate, ambient illumination, the pupils will be noted to have bilaterally, symmetrically, non-rhythmical unrest or variation in size, usually less than 1 mm in amplitude of variation. This is termed hippus
3. Near synkinesis
   a. With sufficient ambient illumination to allow visualization in the pupils, the , patient is asked to shift fixation from the distant object to a near point, preferably the patient's own forefinger. Equal miosis of both pupils will be noted
   b. After shifting fixation back to the distant object, and maintaining the same ambient illumination, a bright light is placed before one or both eyes and the miosis of the light reflex is noted and compared to the "near" miosis. The "light" miosis will be equal to or greater than the "near" miosis
   c. If a patient demonstrates normal reactions of the pupil to light, there is usually no clinical observation to be gained by testing the near response
4. Psychosensory reflex
   a. While maintaining constant "near" and "light" stimuli, the examiner observes pupillary size with the use of a "startle" stimulus such as a loud noise or pain
   b. The pupils will dilate due to two neural mechanisms
      1) Active sympathetic discharges (stimulate iris dilator muscle)
      2) Inhibition of ocular motor nuclei (relaxation of iris sphincter muscle)
   c. The psychosensory reflex is helpful when demonstrating Horner's syndrome
5. Direct pupillary light reflex
   a. By having the subject fixate on a distant object (thereby obviating the miosis associated with accommodation) and the ambient illumination moderately subdued, the direct pupillary response is noted when a bright light is placed before one eye
   b. The pupil constricts briskly, with a subsequent slow dilation to an intermediate size, followed by a state of pupillary unrest (hippus)
   c. The normalcy of the briskness and the latency of the initial response can be

evaluated by clinical experience, but will be further evaluated by comparison with the fellow eye during the direct light reflex test as well as during the swinging flashlight test (see below)

    d. The amplitudes of the initial constriction and subsequent redilation (pupillary escape) depend upon the ambient illumination and the relative brightness of the test light. These amplitudes are also subject to marked individual variation and are best evaluated by comparison with the fellow eye during the swinging flashlight test

6. Consensual pupillary reflex

    a. Because of the equal distribution (to both third nerves) of the photic information provided by one eye, the fellow pupil will behave in the same manner described above for the direct light reflex

7. Swinging flashlight test (Fig. 8-4)

    a. While maintaining the same test conditions described in testing the direct pupillary light reflex, the examiner projects the light on (for example) the right eye and allows the right to go through the phase of initial constriction to a minimum size and subsequent escape to an intermediate size

    b. At this point the examiner quickly swings the light to the left eye which will begin at the intermediate size and go through the phases of initial constriction to a minimum size and subsequent escape to an intermediate size

    c. As soon as the left pupil redilates to the intermediate size, the light is swung to the right eye and a mental note made of the intermediate (starting) size, the latency and briskness of the response, the minimum size, the latency

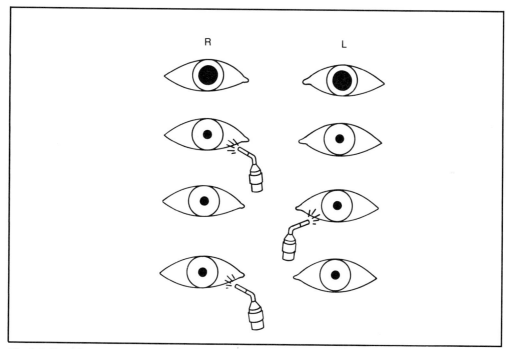

Fig. 8-4. Normal response to swinging flashlight test with no change in size of pupils.

and briskness of the redilation of the intermediate size
d. These characteristics will be exactly the same in both eyes as the light is alternately swung to each eye
e. Key points in proper testing
   1) A bright hand light in a darkened room is essential
   2) The patient should fix on a distant object
   3) The light should cross from one eye to the other fairly rapidly (across the bridge of the nose) and remain three to five seconds on each eye to allow pupillary stabilization

C. Abnormal pupillary states

1. Afferent pupillary defect (Marcus Gunn pupil) (Fig. 8-5)
   a. During the swinging flashlight test, if the amount of light information transmitted from one eye is less than that carried from the fellow eye, the following phenomenon may be noted when the light is swung from the normal eye to the defective eye
      1) Immediate dilation of the pupil, instead of normal initial constriction (3-4+ Marcus Gunn pupil)
      2) No change in pupil size, initially, followed by dilation of the pupils (1-2+ Marcus Gunn pupil)
      3) Initial constriction, but greater escape to a larger intermediate size than when the light is swung back to the normal eye (trace Marcus Gunn pupil)
   b. When the light is swung back to the normal eye, the pupil demonstrates the

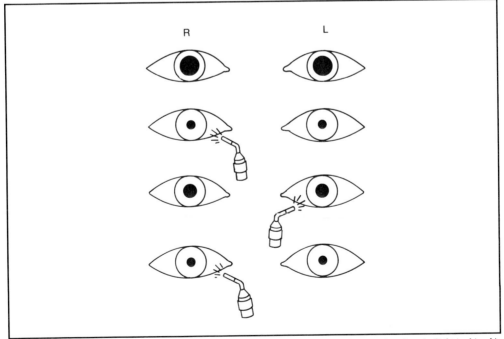

Fig. 8-5. Afferent pupillary defect in left eye using swinging flashlight test. The pupils constrict when the light is shined in the right eye; however, when the flashlight is swung back to the left eye, both pupils dilate.

normal pattern of brisk constriction (of short latency) with subsequent escape to an intermediate size

c. Optic neuropathy (must be unilateral or markedly asymmetric) will usually present with a significant Marcus Gunn pupil

d. Opacities of the ocular media (corneal scar, cataract, vitreous hemorrhage) will not cause a Marcus Gunn pupillary phenomenon if a strong enough flashlight is used

e. Maculopathy, or amblyopic "lazy eye," will not cause a Marcus Gunn phenomenon unless very extensive (less than 20/200 acuity) and then it will only be a 1+ phenomenon, compared to a 3-4+ if the 20/200 acuity were due to an optic neuropathy

f. Extensive retinal damage will cause a significant Marcus Gunn phenomenon

g. Amaurotic pupil: the maximum Marcus Gunn pupil imaginable, seen in patients with "blind eye"

h. There is no such thing as "bilateral" Marcus Gunn pupils; there may be bilaterally reduced direct response of the pupils to light, resulting in "light-near" dissociation, but the Marcus Gunn phenomenon requires asymmetry of the afferent light transmission

i. Isolated, unilateral optic neuropathy does not cause the ipsilateral pupil to be larger; the pupils remain the same size because of the consensual reflex. Unilateral amaurotic mydriasis does not exist!

j. Detection of the afferent pupillary defect requires only one "working" pupil. If one pupil is mechanically or pharmacologically nonreactive, one can simply perform a swinging flashlight test observing the reactive pupil. If the abnormal eye is the eye with a fixed pupil, then the pupil of the normal eye will constrict briskly when the light is shined directly in it and will dilate when the light is shined in the opposite eye. If the abnormal eye is the eye with the reactive pupil, then the pupil will constrict when light is shined in the opposite eye and will dilate when the light is shined directly in it

2. Adie's tonic pupil syndrome

a. Idiopathic, benign cause of internal ophthalmoplegia

b. 80% unilateral initially; tends to become bilateral at a rate of 4% per year

c. Female predilection (70% vs. 30%)

d. Young adults: 20-40 years of age

e. Dilated pupil with poor to absent light reaction

f. Slow constriction to prolonged near-effort and slow redilation (tonic response) after near effort

g. Most patients initially have accommodative paresis, which usually resolves over several months

h. Primary finding of segmental palsy of iris sphincter muscle

i. Adie's pupil frequently (80% of cases) demonstrates cholinergic supersensitivity to weak pilocarpine solutions (.125% or .10%) and Mecholyl (2.5%)

j. Etiology in most cases unknown. Lesion causing Adie's pupil located in the ciliary ganglion or short posterior ciliary nerves; aberrant regeneration of more numerous fibers innervating ciliary muscle (97%) into those subserving iris sphincter muscle (3%)

    k. Adie's syndrome: pupillary abnormalities occurring in a patient with associated diminished deep tendon reflexes

3. Argyll Robertson pupils
   a. Miotic, irregular pupils
   b. Absence of pupillary light response associated with normal anterior visual pathway function
   c. Brisk pupillary constriction to near stimuli
   d. Poor dilation in the dark and in response to mydriatic agents
   e. Condition is usually bilateral, but is often asymmetric and may be unilateral
   f. Etiology: major consideration is neurosyphilis. Other reported causes include diabetes mellitus, chronic alcoholism, multiple sclerosis, sarcoidosis
   g. Site of lesion: most likely in the region of the Sylvian aqueduct in the rostral midbrain interfering with the light reflex fibers and supranuclear inhibitory fibers as they approach the EW nuclei. More ventrally located fibers for near response are spared (Fig. 8-2)

4. Light-near dissociation of the pupils
   a. Better pupillary response to "near" and to "light"
   b. Differential diagnosis
      1) Optic neuropathy or severe retinopathy (probably most common cause)
      2) Adie's tonic pupil
      3) Argyll Robertson pupil
      4) Dorsal midbrain syndrome
      5) Aberrant regeneration of third nerve; defective response to light with aberrent hookup of medial rectus fibers to the pupillary fibers, resulting in pupillary constriction during adduction
      6) Miscellaneous causes: amyloidosis, diabetes, Dejerine-Sottas, Charcot-Marie-Tooth

5. The pupils of coma
   a. Hutchinson pupil
      1) Comatose patient with unilaterally dilated, poorly reactive pupil
      2) Probably due to ipsilateral, expanding, intracranial, supratentorial mass (e.g. tumor, subdural hematoma) that is causing downward displacement of hippocampal gyrus and uncal herniation across the tentorial edge with entrapment of the third nerve (see Fig. 5-4)
      3) The pupillomotor fibers travel in the peripheral portion of the third nerve (near the perineurium) and are subject to early damage from compression
   b. Miosis
      1) During the early stages of coma, the cortical inhibitory input to the EW nucleus is diminished and the pupils are small, but reactive to light

      2) Remember pharmacologic miosis
        a) Morphine
        b) Pilocarpine: if the patient is being incidentally treated for glaucoma
6. The pupils of hospital personnel (pharmacologic blockade)
    a. Unilaterally dilated, fixed pupil
    b. Due to inadvertent contact with mydriatic agent, most commonly atropine
7. Traumatic pupil
    a. Contusion injury of the eye may cause miosis, or mydriasis
    b. Miosis may be due to sphincter spasm seen with iritis
    c. Mydriasis may be due to contusion injury (or actual rupture) of the iris sphincter muscle
      1) Irregular pupil
      2) Poorly responsive to 1% pilocarpine
8. Pharmacologic differentiation of the causes of a fixed, dilated pupil
    a. The patient is tested first with 0.1% pilocarpine, and then, if necessary 1% pilocarpine
    b. If the pupil constricts to 0.1% pilocarpine, then the patient has Adie's pupil; if there is no response to 0.1% pilocarpine, then proceed to 1%
    c. If 1% pilocarpine constricts the involved pupil, then the patient may have a third nerve paresis
    d. If 1% pilocarpine fails to constrict the involved pupil, or does so poorly, the patient has either pharmacological arcade or a traumatic pupil
9. Horner's syndrome (oculosympathetic paralysis)
    a. Three neuron pathways (see Fig. 8-3)
    b. Clinical signs
      1) Miosis of the affected pupil, which is more marked in dim illumination (evoking dilation) than in bright illumination
      2) Ptosis of the upper lid; usually 2-3 mm
      3) Upside-down ptosis of the low lid (due to paresis of inferior tarsal muscle) causing the lower lid to rest 1-2 mm higher on the affected side
      4) Apparent enophthalmos due to narrow palpebral fissure
      5) Anhydrosis of the affected side of the face. This occurs only if the lesion involves the sympathetic pathway proximal to the bifurcation of the common carotid artery, since the sudomotor fibers travel with the external carotid artery
      6) Heterochromia of the affected iris. Characteristic of congenital Horner's with the affected eye having a lighter color
      7) Transient findings
        a) Dilated conjunctival and facial vessels
        b) Decreased intraocular pressure
        c) Increased accommodation
   c. Diagnostic steps in suspected Horner's syndrome
      1) Amount of anisocoria should increase in dim vs. bright illumination. If this step seem inconclusive, then proceed to cocaine test
      2) Cocaine test

          a) Cocaine (4%-10%) eye drops creating sympathomimetic effect by blocking the receptors of norepinephrine at the myoneural junction, thereby prolonging the action of norepinephrine upon the dilator muscle

          b) Therefore, cocaine requires release of norepinephrine at the myoneural junction by a normal functioning oculosympathetic pathway

          c) Cocaine drops result in dilation of the normal pupil

          d) If there is a lesion involving any of the three neurons, pupillary inequality will increase, and the presence of Horner's syndrome is confirmed

      3) Paredrine test

          a) Paredrine (1% hydroxyamphetamine) eye drops create a sympathomimetic effect by causing release of norepinephrine from the nerve endings at the myoneural junction, thereby stimulating the dilator muscle

          b) Paredrine requires that the third order (post-ganglionic) neuron be intact and have normal axoplasmic activity, including formation and transfer of norepinephrine to the nerve ending at the myoneural junction

          c) Paredrine drops result in dilation of the normal pupil

          d) If there is a lesion of the third order neuron, there will be subnormal dilation of the pupil by Paredrine

          e) Pupillary dilation to Paredrine drops will be normal if the Horner's syndrome is due to lesions of the first or second order neurons

      4) Therefore, cocaine serves to confirm the presence of Horner's syndrome and Paredrine serves to identify Horner's due to lesions of the third order neuron

    d. Differentiation of causes of Horner's syndrome

      1) First order neuron lesion (brainstem and spinal cord)

          a) Cerebrovascular accident (Wallenberg's syndrome)

          b) Neck trauma

          c) Neoplasm

          d) Demyelinating disease

          e) Syringomyelia

      2) Second order neuron lesion (preganglionic)

          a) Chest lesions: occult carcinoma of the lung apex (Pancoast's tumor), mediastinal mass, cervical rib

          b) Neck lesions: trauma, abscess, thyroid neoplasm, lymphadenopathy

          c) Surgery: thyroidectomy, radical neck surgery, carotid angiography (direct carotid puncture)

      3) Third order neuron lesion (postganglionic)

          a) Lesion may be extracranial (similar etiologies as listed for second order neuron neck lesions) or cause may be intracranial

b) Migraine variants: cluster headaches, Raeder's paratrigeminal neuralgia
c) Complicated otitis media
d) Cavernous sinus/superior orbital fissure lesion
e) Internal carotid artery dissection
f) Carotid-cavernous fistula
g) Nasopharyngeal carcinoma

D. Evaluation of patient wtih anisocoria

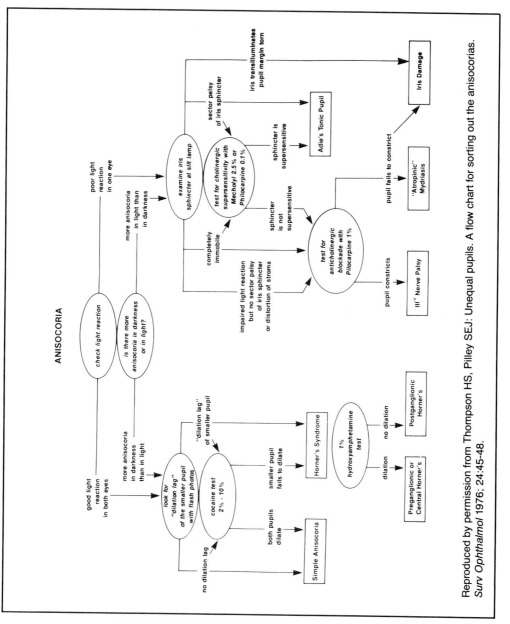

Reproduced by permission from Thompson HS, Pilley SEJ: Unequal pupils. A flow chart for sorting out the anisocorias. *Surv Ophthalmol* 1976; 24:45-48.

123

Bibliography

CHAPTERS

Burde RM, Savino PJ, Trobe JD: Clinical Decisions in Neuroophthalmology. St. Louis, CV Mosby, 1985, Chapter 7, pp. 221-245.

Glaser JS: Neuro-ophthalmology, in Duane TD (ed): Clinical Ophthalmology. Hagerstown, Harper & Row, 1978, Vol. 2, Chapter 15.

Miller NR: Walsh and Hoyt's Clinical Neuro-ophthalmology. Baltimore, Williams & Wilkins, 1985, Chapter 28, 31, pp. 400-441, 469-556.

ARTICLES

Czarnecki JSC, Thompson HS: The iris sphincter in aberrant regeneration of the third nerve. Arch Ophthalmol 1978; 96:1606-1610.

Grimson BS, Thompson HS: Drug testing in Horner's syndrome, in Smith JL, Glaser JS (eds): Neuro-ophthalmology, Symposium of the University of Miami, CV Mosby, St. Louis, Vol. 8, 1975, pp. 265-270.

Keane JR: Oculosympathetic paresis. Arch Neurol 1979; 36:13-15.

Levitan P: Pupillary escape in disease of the retina or optic nerve. Arch Ophthalmol 1959; 62:768-779.

Loewenfeld IE: "Simple, central" anisocoria: A common condition, seldom recognized. Trans Am Acad Ophthalmol Otolaryngol 1977; 83:832-839.

Loewenfeld IE: The Argyll Robertson pupil, 1869-1969. A critical survey of the literature. Surv Ophthalmol 1969; 14:199-299.

Thompson HS: Afferent pupillary defects: pupillary findings associated with defects of the afferent arm of the pupillary light reflex. Am J Ophthalmol 1966; 62:860-873.

Thompson HS: Adie's syndrome: some new observations. Trans Am Ophthalmol Soc 1977; 75:587-626.

Thompson HS: Diagnosing Horner's syndrome. Trans Am Acad Ophthalmol Otolaryngol 1977; 82:OP840-848.

Thompson HS, Newsome DA, Lowenfeld IE: The fixed dilated pupil: sudden iridoplegia or mydriatic drops? A simple diagnostic test. Arch Ophthalmol 1971; 86:21-27.

Thompson HS, Pilley SEJ: Unequal pupils. A flow chart for sorting out the anisocorias. Surv Ophthalmol 1976; 21:45-48.

9

The Swollen Optic Disc

A. Definitions

1. Optic disc edema, swollen disc, "choked" disc: general terms used to describe the optic nerve head affected by a variety of local and systemic causes (Table 9-1)
2. Papilledema: edema of the optic discs due to increased intracranial pressure being transmitted to the optic nerves by the cerebrospinal fluid in the subarachnoid space

B. Pathophysiology of optic disc edema

1. Axonal transport along ganglion cell axons that form the optic nerve occurs in orthograde (cell body to lateral geniculate nucleus) and retrograde (geniculate nucleus to cell body) direction
   a. Orthograde—slow component (1-4 mm/day)
   b. Orthograde—fast component (400 mm/day)
   c. Retrograde (200 mm/day)
2. Accumulation of axoplasmic flow, especially slow orthograde component, at the lamina cribrosa produces disc swelling and nerve fiber layer opacification
3. In papilledema, increased perineural pressure results in damming of the axoplasmic transport. Other causes of interrupted axonal transport include inflammation (e.g. papillitis) and ischemia (e.g. ischemic optic neuropathy)
4. Secondary associated phenomena include dilated retinal veins, exudates, hemorrhages, cotton-wool spots (microinfarcts of the nerve fiber layer)

C. Papilledema

1. Ophthalmoscopic features
   a. Bilateral disc edema (may be asymmetric; rarely unilateral)
   b. Opacification of peripapillary nerve fiber layer
   c. Hyperemia of disc (superficial capillary telangiectasias)
   d. Absent venous pulsations (if venous pulsations are present then the CSF pressure is probably less than 200 mm of water; 20% of normal patients have absent venous pulsations; therefore, the phenomenon of venous pulsations is helpful only if present)
   e. Splinter hemorrhages (i.e. hemorrhages within the nerve fiber layer)
   f. Exudates
   g. Cotton-wool spots
   h. Haziness of the retinal vessels at the disc margins due to swelling of the

125

TABLE 9-1

CAUSES OF OPTIC DISC EDEMA

Ocular Disease	Disc Tumors
Uveitis	Hemangioma
Hypotony	Glioma
Vein occlusion	Metastatic
Metabolic	Vascular
Dysthyroidism	Ischemic neuropathy
Juvenile diabetes	Arteritis, cranial
Proliferative retinopathies	Arteritis, collagen
Inflammatory	Orbital Tumors
Papillitis	Perioptic meningioma
Neuroretinitis	Glioma
Papillophlebitis	Sheath "cysts"
Infiltrative	Retrobulbar mass
Lymphoma	Elevated Intracranial Pressure
Reticuloendothelial	Mass lesion
Systemic Disease	Pseudotumor cerebri
Anemia	Hypertension
Hypoxemia	
Hypertension	

Modified from Glaser JS: Neuro-ophthalmology, in Duane TD: Clinical Ophthalmology. Hagerstown, Harper & Row, 1978, Vol. 2, Chapter 5, p. 23.

     nerve fiber layer, in which the retinal vessels course
- i. Circumferential retinal folds (Paton's lines) in peripapillary region
- j. Obliterated central cup—usually a late finding in papilledema
2. Diagnosis of papilledema constitutes a medical emergency
  - a. Cranial CT scanning to rule out mass lesion
  - b. If no mass discovered and the ventricles are not dilated, CSF analysis to measure opening pressure and look carefully for infectious, infiltrative, or neoplastic cause
3. Visual loss in chronic papilledema
  - a. Enlarged blind spots on visual field examination
  - b. Transient obscurations of vision, unilateral or bilateral "blacking out" or "graying out" of vision, lasting 10 to 15 seconds, and recurring many times per day; often precipitated by sudden changes in posture
  - c. Gradually, progressive visual field loss, usually beginning nasally, and leading to generalized constriction
  - d. Chronic atrophic papilledema with eventual loss of central acuity

D. Pseudotumor Cerebri
    1. Four criteria

          a. Increased intracranial pressure

          b. Normal or small-sized ventricles by CT scanning

          c. Normal CSF composition

          d. Papilledema

    2. Patients may complain of headache, transient visual obscurations, diplopia

    3. In addition to papilledema ophthalmologic findings may include

          a. Sixth nerve palsy (see VI^2 syndrome in Chapter 4)

          b. Visual field changes (large blind spots, generalized constriction)

    4. Patients are frequently young adult, obese females who otherwise report a sense of well-being and have a normal neurologic examination

    5. Recognized etiologies of pseudotumor cerebri (Table 9-2)

E. Papillitis

    1. Primary inflammation of the optic nerve

    2. Two clinical forms of optic neuritis:

          a. Papillitis—intraocular form in which disc swelling is present

          b. Retrobulbar neuritis—optic disc appears normal and inflammatory lesion along course of optic nerve behind globe

    3. Acute impairment of vision

    4. Usually unilateral, although may be bilateral, especially in children

    5. Pain: periocular, retrobulbar, tenderness of the globe, pain especially with eye movement

    6. Afferent pupillary defect present if optic neuritis is unilateral

    7. Visual field defects: usually central scotoma, but may be centrocecal or nerve fiber bundle defects

    8. Cells in vitreous with papillitis

    9. Chronological pattern of visual loss: rapid decrease in acuity during the first two or three days; stable level of decreased vision for seven to ten days; then gradual improvement of vision, frequently returning to normal level within two to three months

    10. Etiologies of optic neuritis

          a. Idiopathic

          b. Multiple sclerosis

          c. Viral infections: childhood (e.g. mumps, measles, chicken pox) adult (e.g. zoster)

          d. Post-viral syndrome

          e. Intraocular inflammation

          f. Contiguous inflammation (e.g. meninges, orbit, sinuses)

          g. Systemic illness (e.g. sarcoid, syphilis, tuberculosis)

    11. Treatment of optic neuritis is controversial; best data suggest steroid therapy (periocular, systemic) may hasten natural course of disease but no proven benefit in ultimate level of visual function (acuity, pupillary reaction, visual field)

F. Ischemic optic neuropathy (ION)

    1. Ischemic infarction of the anterior portion of the optic nerve

    2. Acute visual loss, usually in patients over the age of 60

TABLE 9-2
CONDITIONS ASSOCIATED WITH PSEUDOTUMOR CEREBRI

1. Obstruction or impairment of intracranial venous drainage.
   Dural sinus thrombosis
   Radical neck surgery
   Chronic respiratory insufficiency
   Mediastinal mass

2. Endocrine and Metabolic Dysfunction
   Eclampsia   Diabetic keratoacidosis
   Hypoparathyroidism   Menarche
   Addison's disease   Obesity
   Scurvy   Menstrual abnormalities
   Oral progestational agents   Pregnancy

3. Exogenously Administered Agents
   Heavy metals: lead, arsenic   Nalidixic acid
   Vitamin A   Prolonged steroid therapy
   Tetracycline   Steroid withdrawal

4. Systemic Illness
   Chronic uremia
   Infectious disease
   Bacterial: SBE, meningitis
   Viral: meningitis, Guillain-Barré syndrome
   Parasitic: trypanosomiasis, torulosis
   Neoplastic disease
      Carcinomatous meningitis
      Leukemia
      Spinal cord tumors
   Hematologic disease
      Infectious mononucleosis
      Anemia
      Hemophilia
      Idiopathic thrombocytopenic purpura
   Miscellaneous
      Lupus erythematosus
      Sarcoidosis
      Syphilis
      Paget's disease
      Whipple's disease

3. Clinical settings in which ION is seen
    a. Arterial Disease
        Arteritis
            Cranial Arteritis
            Collagen Diseases
            Syphilis
            Herpes Zoster
        "Arteriosclerosis"—Idiopathic
        Diabetes Mellitus
        Malignant Hypertension
        Migraine
    b. Hypotension/Hypovolemia
        Massive Blood Loss
        Cardiac Insufficiency
        Surgical Hypotension
        Anemia
    c. Other
        Post-Cataract Surgery
4. Differential diagnosis involves arteritis (giant cell arteritis) vs. idiopathic ("arteriosclerotic") as major causes of ischemic optic neuropathy
5. Characteristics of Ischemic Optic Neuropathy

	Idiopathic ("Arteriosclerotic")	Cranial Arteritis
Age Peak	60-70 years	70-80 years
Visual loss	Minimal to severe	Usually severe
Involvement of second eye	Approximately 40%	Approximately 75%
Acute Fundus	Swollen disc	Swollen disc, may be pallid
Other ophthalmologic presentations	—	Central retinal artery occlusion; choroidal infarction; anterior segment ischemia
Systemic	Hypertension (approximately 50%)	Headache, malaise, weakness, weight loss, jaw pain, polymyalgia
ESR (Westergren) (mm/hr.)	Up to 40	Usually high (50-120)
Response to steroids	None	Relief of systemic symptoms; infrequent return to vision; protect other eye

Modified from Glaser J.S.: Neuro-ophthalmology, in Duane TD: Clinical Ophthalmology, Hagerstown, Harper & Row, 1978, Vol. 2, Chapter 5, p. 26.

6. ION is virtually always accompanied by disc swelling in the acute stage; rare exception in retrobulbar ischemic optic neuropathy associated with giant cell arteritis
7. Visual defect is usually maximal in onset. On occasion field abnormality may progress within the first month. Subsequent improvement in vision is rare
8. Recognition of cases due to giant cell arteritis is essential; prompt steroid therapy may restore some degree of vision, avert visual loss in the fellow eye, and improve long-term systemic morbidity and mortality

G. Miscellaneous causes of swollen optic disc

1. Orbital disease: optic nerve or arachnoid cyst, orbital tumor, ocular dysthyroidism
2. Intraocular disease: uveitis, vein occlusion, disc tumor, hypotony
3. Diabetic papillopathy
   a. Usually occurs in teenager with more than 10 year history of insulin-dependent diabetes
   b. Usually bilateral but may be unilateral
   c. May be relatively asymptomatic or a patient may experience significant acuity and visual field loss
   d. Visual acuity usually improves within three months and prognosis is generally, but not uniformly, favorable
4. Papillophlebitis (retinal vasculitis, optic disc vasculitis, "big blind spot" syndrome)
   a. Usually unilateral disc edema
   b. Young, healthy adults
   c. Vague visual complaints of blurred vision with minimal impairment of acuity (usually no worse than 20/30)
   d. No afferent pupillary defect
   e. Only visual field abnormality is enlargement of blind spot
   f. Disc swelling with associated engorged retinal veins and occasional retinal hemorrhages
   g. Spontaneous, usually complete recovery within several months to one year
   h. Pathologic examination reveals inflammation of the retinal veins, although etiology of inflammation is unknown
5. Leber's optic neuropathy (Table 10-1)
   a. Most often, but not exclusively, affects males in the second or third decade of life
   b. Rapid monocular visual loss to a variable level (20/200 or worse)
   c. Second eye usually affected within days or weeks
   d. In acute phase, optic disc may appear normal or have typical triad of findings
      1) Circumpapillary telangiectatic microangiopathy
      2) Prominent nerve fiber layer around disc
      3) Absence of dye leakage from the disc or peripapillary region with fluorescein angiography
   e. Visual field abnormality is centrocecal scotoma

      f. Ultimately the patient develops either temporal or generalized disc pallor

      g. Hereditary pattern of Leber's optic neuropathy unknown but

           1) Affected male does not transmit the disease or the carrier state to his offspring

           2) The heterozygous female may transmit the disease to sons and the carrier state to daughters

           3) Look for family history in brothers or maternal uncles

      h. No effective treatment

   6. Spheno-orbital meningioma

      a. Chronic compression of the intraorbital or intracanalicular optic nerve

      b. Clinical triad

           1) Visual loss

           2) Optic disc swelling that resolves into optic atrophy

           3) Appearance of optociliary shunt vessels

      c. The clinical picture may be seen with optic nerve glioma, chronic papilledema, craniopharyngioma

H. Pseudopapilledema (anomalous elevation of the discs; congenitally full discs)

   1. Ophthalmoscopic features

      a. Disc is not hyperemic, and there are no dilated capillaries on its surface

      b. Despite disc elevation, surface arteries are not obscured (no peripapillary nerve fiber layer opacification)

      c. Physiologic cup usually absent

      d. May see anomalous branching and tortuosity of retinal vessels (abnormally large number of branches at disc margin)

      e. May see hyaline bodies or drusen buried in disc of patient or relatives

      f. No hemorrhages (rare exceptions)

      g. No exudates or cotton-wool spots

      h. Disc usually has irregular border with pigment epithelial defects in peripapillary retina

      i. Visual field testing may show enlarged blind spots and nerve fiber bundle defects

   2. If exam suggestive of buried disc drusen, may use orbital ultrasonography or CT to "visualize" them

Bibliography

BOOKS

Hayreh SS: Anterior ischemic optic neuropathy. New York, Springer-Verlag, 1975.

Healey LA, Wilske KR: The systemic manifestations of temporal arteritis. New York, Grune & Stratton, 1978.

CHAPTERS

Glaser JS: Neuro-ophthalmology, in Duane TD (ed.): Clinical Ophthalmology. Hagerstown, Harper & Row, 1978, Vol. 2, Chapter 5.

Miller NR: Walsh and Hoyt's Clinical Neuro-ophthalmology. Baltimore, Williams & Wilkins, 1985, Chapters 12-18, pp. 175-270.

ARTICLES

Appen RE, deVenecia G, Ferwerda J: Optic disc vasculitis. Am J Ophthalmol 1980; 90:352-359.

Barr CC, Glaser JS, Blankenships G: Acute disc swelling in juvenile diabetes. Clinical profile and natural history of 12 cases. Arch Ophthalmol 1980; 92:2185-2192.

Bird AC: Is there a place for corticosteroids in the treatment of optic neuritis? In Brockhurst RM, Borchoff SA, Hutchinson BT, et al (eds): Controversy in ophthalmology. Philadelphia, WB Saunders, 1977, Chapter 28, pp. 822-829.

Boghen DR, Glaser JS: Ischemic optic neuropathy. The clinical profile and natural history. Brain 1975; 98:689-708.

Cogan DG: Blackouts not obviously due to carotid occlusion. Arch Ophthalmol 1961; 66:180-187.

Cohen MM, Lendl S, Wolf PA: A prospective study of the risk of developing multiple sclerosis in uncomplicated optic neuritis. Neurology 1979; 29:208-213.

Corbett JJ, Savino PJ, Thompson HS, et al: Visual loss in pseudotumor cerebrei. Follow-up of 57 patients from five to 41 years and a profile of 14 patients with permanent severe visual loss. Arch Neurol 1982; 39:461-474.

Frisén L, Hoyt WF, Tengroth BM: Optociliary veins, disc pallor, and visual loss: a triad of signs indicating spheno-orbital meningioma. Acta Ophthalmol 1973; 51:241-249.

Hayreh MS, Hayreh SS: Optic disc edema in raised intracranial pressure: I. Evaluation and resolution. Arch Ophthalmol 1977; 95:1237-1244.

Hayreh SS, Hayreh MS: Optic disc edema in raised intracranial pressure: II. Early detection with fluorescein fundus angiography and stereoscopic color photography. Arch Ophthalmol 1977; 95:1245-1254.

Hayreh SS: Optic disc edema in raised intracranial pressure: V. Pathogenesis. Arch Ophthalmol 1977; 95:1553-1565.

Hayreh SS: Optic disc edema in raised intracranial pressure: VI. Associated visual disturbances and their pathogenesis. Arch Ophthalmol 1977; 1566-1579.

Hayreh SS: Optic disc vasculitis. Brit J Ophthalmol 1972; 56:652-670.

Levin BE: The clinical significance of spontaneous pulsations of the retinal vein. Arch Neurol 1978; 35:37-40.

Lonn LI, Hoyt WF: Papillophlebitis: a cause of protracted yet benign optic disc edema. Eye Ear Nose Throat Monthly 1966; 45:62-68.

Miller GR, Smith JL: Ischemic optic neuropathy. Am J Ophthalmol 1966; 62:103-115.

Minkler DS, Tso MOM, Zimmerman LE: A light microscopic, autoradiographic study of axoplasmic transport in the optic nerve head during ocular hypotony, increased intracranial pressure, and papilledema. Am J Ophthalmol 1976; 82:741-759.

Okun E: Chronic papilledema simulating hyaline bodies of the optic disc. Am J Ophthalmol 1962; 53:922-927.

Rosenberg MA, Savino PJ, Glaser JS: A clinical analysis of pseudopapilledema: I. Population, laterality, acuity, refractive error, ophthalmoscopic characteristics, and coincident disease. Arch Ophthalmol 1979; 97:65-70.

Rush JA: Pseudotumor cerebrei: clinical profile and visual outcome in 63 patients. Mayo Clin Proc 1980; 55:541-546.

Savino PJ, Glaser JS, Rosenburg MA: A clinical analysis of pseudopapilledema: II. Visual field defects. Arch Ophthalmol 1979; 97:71-75.

Smith JL, Hoyt WF, Susac JO: Ocular fundus in acute Leber's optic neuropathy. Arch Ophthalmol 1973; 90:349-354.

Spencer WH: Drusen of the optic disc and aberrant axoplasmic transport. The XXIII Edward Jackson Memorial Lecture. Am J Ophthalmol 1978; 85:1-12.

Trobe JD, Glaser JS, Laflamme P: Dysthyroid optic neuropathy: clinical profile and rationale for management. Arch Ophthalmol 1978; 96:1199-1209.

Tso MO, Hayreh SS: Optic disc edema in raised intracranial pressure: III. A pathologic study of experimental papilledema. Arch Ophthalmol 1977; 95:1448-1457.

Tso MOM, Hayreh SS: Optic disc edema in raised intracranial pressure: IV. Axoplasmic transport in experimental papilledema. Arch Ophthalmol 1977; 95:1458-1462.

Weisberg LA: Benign intracranial hypertension. Medicine 1975; 54:197-207.

Wirtschafter JD, Rizzo FJ, Smiley BC: Optic nerve axoplasm and papilledema. Surv Ophthalmol 1975; 20:157-189.

Wise GN, Henkind P, Alterman M: Optic disc drusen and subretinal hemorrhage. Trans Am Acad Ophthalmol Otolaryngol 1974; 78:212-219.

The Pale Optic Disc—Optic Atrophy

A. Optic disc pallor vs. optic atrophy
  1. Ophthalmoscopic appearance of disc pallor alone does not establish the presence of optic atrophy
  2. Frequently the temporal side of the normal disc has less color than the nasal side
  3. Optic atrophy is a pathologic description of optic nerve shrinkage from any process that produces degeneration of axons in the anterior visual system (retinogeniculate) pathway
  4. The clinical diagnosis of optic atrophy is based on
     a. Ophthalmoscopic abnormalities of color and structure of the disc with associated changes in retinal vessels and nerve fiber layer
     b. Defective visual function (acuity, color vision, pupils, fields, visual evoked response) and can be localized to the optic nerve

B. Histopathologic considerations
  1. When a visual axon is severed, its ascending (to the brain) segment disintegrates and disappears in approximately seven days. This is termed Wallerian degeneration
  2. The portion of the axon still connected to the ganglion cell body remains viable for three to four weeks but then rapidly degenerates by six to eight weeks. This is called descending (to the eye) degeneration
  3. With the completion of descending degeneration of axons, optic disc pallor appears. Currently there are two major theories to explain acquired disc pallor
     a. Vascular-glial theory: When the optic nerve degenerates its blood supply is reduced, and smaller vessels, recognizable in the normal disc, disappear from view. In addition, formation of glial tissue at the nerve head is said to occur with optic atrophy
     b. Nerve fiber layer theory (Fig. 10-1): With degeneration of visual axons, there is alteration in the thickness and cytoarchitecture of nerve fiber bundles passing between glial columns containing capillaries. Alteration of light conducted along the nerve fiber bundles leads to the appearance of pallor, and there is no reduction in blood supply to the optic disc

135

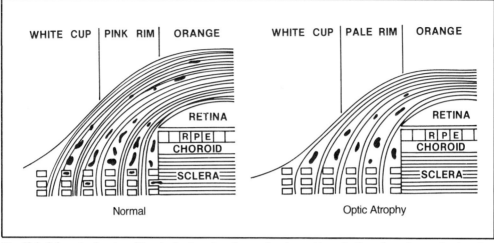

Fig. 10-1. Schematic drawing of longitudinal section of normal and atrophic optic discs. In optic atrophy there is a decrease in the number of nerve fibers and capillaries, but the proportion of capillaries per unit volume is unchanged. (Redrawn from Quigley HA, Anderson DR: The histologic basis of optic disk pallor in experimental optic atrophy. Am J Ophthalmol 1977; 83:709-717).

C. Ophthalmoscopic features of optic atrophy

1. As a general rule, fundus signs are not specific for any particular etiology of optic atrophy, and the diagnosis must be obtained from non-ophthalmoscopic findings
2. In the early stages of atrophy, the optic disc loses its reddish hue, and the substance of the disc slowly melts away to leave a pale, shallow concave meniscus, the exposed lamina cribrosa
3. Ipsilateral attenuation of the retinal arterioles is frequently a sign of old central retinal artery occlusion
4. Healed papillitis or ischemic optic neuropathy may cause narrowing of retinal arterioles only in their peripapillary segment, after which they appear to enlarge slightly in caliber as they traverse the fundus ("reverse taper sign")
5. Pathologic disc cupping may develop along with disc pallor in patients without glaucoma. Etiologies include ischemia, compression, inflammation, and trauma
6. Nerve fiber layer defects should be carefully looked for when suspecting optic atrophy. They apper as dark slits or wedges and are most easily identified in the superior and inferior arcuate regions where the nerve fiber layer is particularly thick. Also, vessels in this area, having lost their surrounding nerve fiber covering, appear darker than normal and stand out sharply
7. "Bow-tie" or "band" optic atrophy
   a. Specific patterns of nerve fiber layer and optic atrophy from optic chiasmal and retrochiasmal-pregeniculate lesions
   b. With temporal field defects, loss of nerve fiber from ganglion cells nasal to fovea
   c. Results in atrophy of nasal and temporal portions of the disc, with relative

sparing of superior and inferior arcuate bundles
d. Arcuate bundles spared since they arise from ganglion cells both temporal and nasal to disc
8. Homonymous hemioptic (hemianopic) hypoplasia
a. Optic disc findings in patients with congenital cerebral hemiatrophy, presumably due to fetal vascular insufficiency
b. Fundus ipsilateral to hemispheric defect shows slightly small optic disc with temporal pallor and loss of nerve fiber layer of ganglion cells temporal to fovea
c. Fundus contralateral to hemispheric defect shows small disc with "band" atrophy
d. Associated findings include mental retardation, seizures, congenital hemiplegia and complete homonymous hemianopia

D. The hereditary optic neuropathies
1. These forms of optic nerve disease cause insidious, bilateral, symmetric loss of central acuity
2. Table 10-1 summarizes the major forms of hereditary optic nerve disease

E. Toxic and deficiency optic neuropathies
1. Particular forms of medical therapy or exposure to specific toxins may lead to bilateral retrobulbar optic neuropathy, characterized by visual loss, severe dyschromatopsia, central field defects with occasional peripheral field constriction, and initially normal-appearing optic discs that may gradually become pale
2. Frequently used drugs that may cause optic atrophy include
a. Ethambutol
b. Isoniazid
c. Chloramphenicol
d. Streptomycin
e. Digitalis
f. Chloroquine
g. Placidyl
h. Chlorpropamide
3. Grant's Toxicology of the Eye lists over 20 toxins associated with optic neuropathy, including
a. Arsenic
b. Lead
c. Hexachlorophene (PhisoHex)
d. Lead
e. Lysol
f. Quinine
4. Deficiency optic neuropathies
a. Clinical picture of progressive bilateral visual loss, with central or centrocecal scotomas and some degree of temporal disc pallor and atrophy of the papillomacular nerve fiber layer

        b. Vitamin deficiencies that may be responsible for optic atrophy include
            1) Vitamin B12 (cobalamin)
            2) Vitamin B6 (pyridoxine)
            3) Vitamin B1 (thiamine)
            4) Niacin
            5) Vitamin B2 (riboflavin)
            6) Folic acid

5. Tobacco-Alcohol amblyopia
    a. Similar clinical picture to deficiency optic neuropathies listed above
    b. Continuing controversy as to whether this represents a form of toxic (cyanide) or deficiency (vitamin) optic nerve disease
    c. In general, prognosis for recovery of vision is good except in the most chronic cases

F. Infiltrative Optic Neuropathy

1. Optic disc initially swollen or normal; ultimately becomes pale
2. Often acute visual loss
3. Etiology may be benign or malignant
    a. sarcoidosis
    b. lymphoma
    c. leukemia
    d. plasmacytoma
    e. malignant histocytosis

G. Carcinomatous Optic Neuropathy

1. Fundus typically normal at onset of visual loss, with disc gradually becoming pale
2. Patient may or may not have history of known malignancy
3. Optic neuropathy may be isolated or accompanied by other neurologic defects
4. Visual loss typically acute and devastating
5. Unless large intraparenchymal CNS spread has occurred, radiologic studies (CT, MRI, angiography) will be normal
6. Due to microscopic infiltrates of nerve and its sheaths

H. Radiation Optic Neuropathy

1. Due to delayed cerebral radionecrosis of optic nerve and chiasm
2. Follows radiation therapy for perisellar tumor such as pituitary adenoma, craniopharyngioma, invasive sinus carcinoma
3. Diagnostic criteria
    a. acute visual loss (monocular or binocular)
    b. visual field defects indicating optic nerve or chiasmal dysfunction
    c. absence of optic disc edema
    d. onset usually within three years of therapy (peak: 1-1½ years)
    e. no CT evidence of anterior visual pathway compression
4. Pathology: fibrinoid necrosis of blood vessels, demyelination, necrosis
5. Treatment: none of proven efficacy

Table 10-1

Heredofamilial Optic Atrophies

	Dominant	Recessive			Indeterminate
	Juvenile (Infantile)	Early infantile (Congenital); Simple	Behr's type; Complicated	With diabetes mellitus; ± deafness	Leber's disease
Age at onset	Childhood (4 to 8 years)	Early childhood† (3 to 4 years)	Childhood (1 to 9 years)	Childhood (6 to 14 years)	Early adulthood (18 to 30 years; up to sixth decade)
Visual impairment	Mild / moderate (20 / 40 - 20 / 200)	Severe (20 / 200 - HM)	Moderate (20 / 200)	Severe (20 / 400 - FC)	Moderate / severe (20 / 200 - FC)
Nystagmus	Rare‡	Usual	In 50%	Absent	Absent
Optic disc	Mild temporal pallor; ± temporal excavation	Marked diffuse pallor (± arteriolar attenuation) ϕ	Mild temporal pallor	Marked diffuse pallor	Moderate diffuse pallor; disc swelling in acute phase
Color vision	Blue-yellow dyschromatopsia	Severe dyschromatopsia / achromatopsia	Moderate to severe dyschromatopsia	Severe dyschromatopsia	Dense central scotoma for colors
Course	Variable, slight progression	Stable	Stable	Progressive	Acute visual loss, then usually stable; may improve / worsen

HM, hand motions; FC, finger counting.

† Difficult to assess in infancy, but visual impairment usually manifests by age 4 years.

‡ Presence of nystagmus with poor vision and earlier onset suggests separate congenital or infantile form.

ϕ Distinguished from tapetoretinal degenerations by normal electroretinogram (ERG).

From Glaser JS: Heredofamilial disorders of the optic nerve. In Renie WA (ed): Goldberg's Genetic and Metabolic Eye Disease. Boston; Little Brown, 1974.

Bibliography

CHAPTERS

Glaser JS: Heredofamilial disorders of the optic nerve, In Goldberg MF (ed): Genetic and metabolic eye disease. Boston, Little Brown & Co., 1974, Chapter 19, pp. 463-486.

Miller NR: Walsh and Hoyt's Clinical Neuro-Ophthalmology. Baltimore, Williams & Wilkins, 1985, Chapter 24, pp. 311-328.

ARTICLES

Altrocchi PA, Remhardt PM, Eckman PB: Blindness and meningeal carcinomatosis. Arch Ophthalmol 1972; 88:508-512.

Ellis W, Little HC: Leukemic infiltration of the optic nerve head. Am J Ophthalmol 1973; 75:867-871.

Gudas PP: Optic nerve myeloma. Am J Ophthalmol 1971; 71:1085-1089.

Hoyt WF, Rios-Montenegro EN, Behrens MM, et al: Homonymous hemioptic hypoplasia: Funduscopic features in standard and red-free illumination in three patients with congenital hemiplegia. Br J Ophthalmol 1972; 56:537-545.

Jampol LM, Woodfin W, McLean ED: Optic nerve sarcoidosis: report of a case. Arch Ophthalmol 1972; 87:355-360.

Kline LB, Garcia JH, Harsh GR III: Lymphomatous optic neuropathy. Arch Ophthalmol 1984; 102:1655-1657.

Kline LB, Glaser JS: Dominant optic atrophy: the clinical profile. Arch Ophthalmol 1979; 97:1680-1686.

Kline LB, Kim JY, Ceballos R: Radiation optic neuropathy. Ophthalmology 1985; 92:1118-1126.

Lessell S, Gise RL, Krohel GB: Bilateral optic neuropathy with remission in young man. Variation on a theme by Leber? Arch Neurol 1983; 40:2-6.

Nikoskelainen E, Hoyt WF, Nummelin K: Ophthalmologic findings in Leber's hereditary optic neuropathy. I: Fundus findings in asymptomatic family members. Arch Ophthalmol 1982; 100:1597-1602.

Nikoskelainen E, Hoyt WF, Nummelin K: Ophthalmologic findings in Leber's hereditary optic neuropathy. II. The fundus findings in the affected family member. Arch Ophthalmol 1983; 101:1059-1060.

Nikoskelainen E, Hoyt WF, Nummelin K, et al: Ophthalmologic findings in Leber's hereditary optic neuropathy. III. Fluorescein angiographic studies. Arch Ophthalmol 1984; 102:981-989.

Trobe JD, Glaser JS, Cassady JC: Optic atrophy. Differential diagnosis by fundus observation alone. Arch Ophthalmol 1980; 98:1040-1045.

Trobe JD, Glaser JS, Cassady JC, et al: Non-glaucomatous excavation of the optic disc. Arch Ophthalmol 1980; 98:1046-1050.

Unsöld R, Hoyt WF: Band atrophy of the optic nerve. The histology of temporal hemianopsia. Arch Ophthalmol 1980; 98:1637-1638.

Victor M: Tobacco alcohol amblyopia: A critique of current concepts of this disorder, with special reference to the role of nutritional deficiency in its causation. Arch Ophthalmol 1963; 70:313-318.

Wokes F: Tobacco amblyopia. Lancet 1958; 2:526-527.

11

Myasthenia and Ocular Myopathies

A. These disorders produce ocular motor dysfunction through involvement of the extraocular muscles and the neuromuscular junction. Some of these entities may simulate isolated or combined ocular motor cranial nerve palsies

B. Myasthenia Gravis
  1. Disease characterized clinically by muscle weakness and fatigue
  2. It is the most common disorder affecting the neuromuscular junction
  3. Myasthenia involves skeletal and not visceral musculature; therefore, the pupil and ciliary muscle are unaffected. Major ophthalmologic complaints are ptosis and diplopia
  4. Ocular involvement eventually occurs in 90% of myasthenics, and accounts for the initial complaint in 75%. Approximately 80% of patients with ocular onset progress to involvement of other muscle groups (usually within two years) while 20% have only ocular complaints
  5. Impaired neuromuscular transmission of myasthenia is due to the presence of antibodies to acetylcholine receptors in the motor endplate of striated muscles. This leads to a reduction in the number of acetylcholine receptors
  6. Clinical characteristics of ocular myasthenia
     a. Variability of muscle function within minutes, hours, days or weeks
     b. Remissions and exacerbations (often triggered by infection or trauma)
     c. Onset at any age
     d. Ptosis (unilateral or bilateral) worse at end of day; may "shift" from eye to eye
     e. Extraocular muscle involvement follows no set pattern; any ocular movement pattern may develop and thus mimic any ocular motor cranial nerve palsy or central gaze disturbance (e.g. gaze palsy, INO, gaze-evoked nystagmus)
     f. Dysthyroidism is found in approximately 5% of myasthenics, and also an increased incidence of thymoma, and collagen vascular disorders
  7. Diagnosis of ocular myasthenia
     a. Lid fatigue: with sustained upward gaze ptosis becomes more marked
     b. Lid-twitch sign (Cogan): the patient looks down for 10-15 seconds and is

then asked to rapidly refixate in the primary position. A positive lid-twitch sign consists of an upward overshoot of the lid, which then falls to its previously ptotic position

c. Enhanced ptosis: if ptosis is asymmetric, the patient may use the frontalis muscle to elevate both lids, producing what appears to be lid retraction on one side. If the more ptotic lid is elevated, the previously retracted one will fall

d. Variability in measuring phorias or tropias during the same examination or at different times is very suggestive of myasthenia

e. Myasthenic ptosis is frequently associated with orbicularis weakness

f. Tensilon (edrophonium chloride) test: one positive test establishes the diagnosis of myasthenia, yet myasthenia may exist even in the face of a negative Tensilon test. (See Chapter 15 for correct way to perform a Tensilon test)

g. Acetylcholine receptor antibodies, if present, are diagnostic of myasthenia. However, only about one third of patients with ocular myasthenia have detectable antibody levels

h. Electromyography (EMG): with repetitive supramaximal motor nerve stimulation there is a decremental muscular response in myasthenia. Helpful if present, but may be normal response in clinically uninvolved extremity musculature in patients with ocular myasthenia. Should be performed on orbicularis oculi as well

8. Treatment of ocular myasthenia
   a. Occlusion of one eye
   b. Prism spectacles
   c. Pyridostigmine (Mestinon)
   d. Systemic steroids

C. Chronic progressive external ophthalmoplegia (CPEO)

1. Comprises a group of disorders characterized by insidiously progressive, symmetric immobility of the eyes, with lids typically ptotic, the orbicularis oculi weak, and the pupils spared

2. The eye movements remain limited with doll's head and caloric stimulation

3. CPEO may occur in an isolated ocular form, may have a hereditary pattern or may be part of a recognizable clinical entity
   a. Oculopharyngeal dystrophy: dysphagia, family history of ophthalmoplegia, often French-Canadian ancestry
   b. Kearns-Sayre syndrome: triad of CPEO, cardiac conduction defect, pigmentary retinopathy
   c. Ophthalmoplegia plus: term applied to instances in which CPEO is associated with the above abnormalities "plus" a variety of others including elevated CSF protein, spongiform degeneration of the cerebrum and brainstem, slow EEG, subnormal intelligence, hearing loss

4. Muscle biopsy (ocular or limb) will demonstrate mitochondrial accumulations beneath the plasma membrane and between myofibrils. Using a modified

trichrome stain these abnormal muscle fibers have been called "ragged red" fibers

    5. A condition simulating CPEO is known as Progressive Supranuclear Palsy (PSP) or Steele-Richardson-Olszewski syndrome
        a. Vertical gaze, especially downward gaze, is affected first
        b. Eventually horizontal gaze is involved
        c. Doll's head and caloric testing demonstrate full excursions until late in course of disease
        d. Additional clinical findings: dystonic rigidity of neck and trunk, masked face, dysesthesia, hyperreflexia, dementia
        e. Neurodegenerative condition characterized pathologically by neuronal loss, gliosis, neurofibrillary tangles, and demyelination centered in the brainstem reticular formation and ocular motor nuclei

D. Myotonic dystrophy

    1. Autosomal dominant muscular dystrophy in which myotonia is accompanied by dystrophic changes in other tissues and organs
    2. Myotonia is a phenomenon in which muscle fibers have a pathologically persistent activity after a strong contraction or are continuously active when they should be relaxed
    3. Ophthalmologic signs
        a. Bilateral ptosis
        b. Progressive external ophthalmoplegia
        c. Myotonia of lid closure and gaze holding
        d. Orbicularis weaknesses
        e. Polychromatophilic cataracts
        f. Miotic pupils, sluggish to light and near
        g. Retinal pigmentary degeneration
    4. Multiple systemic findings include face, neck, and limb myopathy with atrophy, testicular atrophy, baldness, myotonic cardiomyopathy

E. Dysthyroid myopathy

    1. A restrictive myopathy occurring commonly in middle-aged and elderly individuals leading to ophthalmoparesis and diplopia
    2. Lymphocytic and plasmacytic infiltration of extraocular muscles, leads to edema, activation of fibroblasts with production of acid mucopolysaccharide and fibrosis
    3. Variety of ocular motility patterns produced
        a. "Elevator palsy" due to fibrotic shortening of the inferior rectus
        b. "Abduction weakness" due to involvement of the medial rectus, mimicking a sixth nerve palsy
        c. Superior and lateral rectus muscles less frequently involved
    4. Additional findings include
        a. Proptosis
        b. Lids: retraction, lid lag on downward gaze (von Graefe's sign), edema
        c. Conjunctiva: injection over horizontal rectus muscles, chemosis

       d. Cornea: keratopathy, erosions, ulceration

       e. Optic neuropathy due to compression at orbital apex by enlarged extra-ocular muscles

    5. Diagnostic studies

       a. Forced duction testing (see Chapter 15)

       b. Ultrasonography to measure size of extraocular muscles

       c. Orbital CT scanning

       d. Thyroid function tests

    6. Association of dysthyroidism with myasthenia; two diseases may coexist and give a variety of ocular findings

F. Idiopathic orbital inflammation (orbital pseudotumor)

    1. A syndrome occurring in any age group consisting of acute onset of orbital pain, chemosis, conjunctival injection and frequently proptosis

    2. If the inflammatory process affects one or more of the extraocular muscles, the term orbital myositis is employed. These patients typically complain of diplopia

    3. Pathologic studies in such cases demonstrate orbital structures (blood vessels, muscles, lacrimal glands, etc.) infiltrated with chronic inflammatory cells

    4. In the vast majority of cases the etiology of the inflammatory response is unknown, although it may occur with systemic disorders including lupus erythematosus, rheumatoid arthritis, sarcoidosis, Wagener's granulomatosis, dermatomyositis

    5. Diagnostic studies

       a. Orbital ultrasonography

       b. Orbital CT scanning

       c. Orbital biopsy

    6. Treatment modalities

       a. Systemic steroids usually produce dramatic improvement in symptoms in 24-48 hours with clearing of signs over 1-4 weeks

       b. Orbital radiation therapy: 1000-2000 rad

       c. Chlorambucil for chronic, recurrent orbital pseudotumor

    7. It may be difficult to distinguish between benign orbital inflammation and orbital lymphoma, both clinically and pathologically. All patients with idiopathic orbital inflammation must be followed carefully. An initial salutory response to steroid therapy by no means excludes a malignant process

Bibliography

BOOKS

Char DH: Thyroid eye disease. Baltimore, Williams & Wilkins, 1985.

Gorman CA, Waller RR, Dyer JA: The Eye and Orbit in Thyroid Disease. New York, Raven Press, 1984.

Lisak RP, Barchi RL: Myasthenia gravis. Philadelphia, WB Saunders, 1982.

CHAPTERS

Daroff RB: Ocular myasthenia: diagnosis and therapy. In Glaser JS (ed): Neuro-ophthalmology. St. Louis, CV Mosby, 1980, Volume 10, Chapter 6, pp. 62-71.

Glaser JS: Neuro-Ophthalmology, in Duane TD: Clinical Ophthalmology. Hagerstown, Harper & Row, 1978, Vol. 2, Chapter 12.

Miller NR: Walsh and Hoyt's Clinical Neuro-ophthalmology. Baltimore, Williams and Wilkins, 1985, Chapter 36, pp. 785-891.

Rowland LP: Progressive external ophthalmoplegia, In Vinken PJ, Bruyn GW, DeJong JMBV (eds): Systemic disorders and atrophies. Part II. Handbook of Clinical Neurology. New York, Elsevier Pub Co., 1975, Vol. 22, pp. 177-202.

ARTICLES

Babel J: Ophthalmological aspects of myotonic dystrophy, In Huber A, Klein D (eds): Neurogenetics and Neuro-ophthalmology. Amsterdam, Elsevier/North-Holland, 1981, pp. 19-30.

Chavis RM, Garner A, Wright JE: Inflammatory orbital pseudotumors. A clinicopathologic study. Arch Ophthalmol 1978; 96:1817-1822.

Cogan DG: Myasthenia gravis: a review of the disease and a description of lid twitch as a characteristic sign. Arch Ophthalmol 1965; 74:217-221.

Daroff RB: Chronic progressive external ophthalmoplegia: a critical review. Arch Ophthalmol 1969; 82:845-850.

Drachman DA: Ophthalmoplegia plus: the neuro-degenerative disorders associated with progressive external ophthalmoplegia. Arch Neurol 1968; 18:654-674.

Drachman DB, Seybold ME: Prednisone schedule for myasthenia gravis. N Engl J Med 1974; 290:631-632.

Dresner SC, Kennerdell JS: Dysthyroid orbitopathy. Neurology 1985; 35:1628-1634.

Glaser JS: Myasthenia pseudo-internuclear ophthalmoplegia. Arch Ophthalmol 1966; 75:363-366.

Gorelick PB, Rosenberg M, Pagano RJ: Enhanced ptosis in myasthenia gravis. Arch Neurol 1981; 38:531.

Kearns TB, Sayre GP: Retinitis pigmentosa, external ophthalmoplegia and complete heart block. Arch Ophthalmol 1958; 60:280-289.

Kennerdell JS, Rosenbaum AE, El-Hosby MH: Apical optic nerve compression of dysthyroid optic neuropathy on computed tomography. Arch Ophthalmol 1981; 99:807-809.

Kennerdall JS, Dresner SC: The nonspecific orbital inflammatory syndromes. Surv Ophthalmol 1984; 29:92-113.

Lessell S, Coppeto J, Samet S: Ophthalmoplegia in myotonic dystrophy. Am J Ophthalmol 1971; 71:1231-1235.

Osher RH: Myasthenia "Oculomotor" palsy. Ann Ophthalmol 1979; 11:31-34.

Osher RH, Glaser JS: Myasthenic sustained gaze fatigue. Am J Ophthalmol 1980; 89:443-445.

Osserman KE, Kaplan LI: Rapid diagnostic test for myasthenia gravis: increased muscle strength, without fasciculations, after intravenous administration of edrophonium (Tensilon) chloride. JAMA 1952; 150:265-269.

Rootman J, Nugent R: The classification and management of acute orbital pseudotumors. Ophthalmology 1982; 89:1040-1048.

Sergott RC, Glaser JS: Grave's ophthalmopathy: a clinical and immunologic review. Surv Ophthalmol 1981; 26:1-21.

Skalka HW: Ultrasonography in the diagnosis of endocrine orbitopathy, In Smith JL (ed): Neuro-Ophthalmology Focus 1980. New York, Masson, 1979, pp. 211-216.

Spoor TC, Martinez AJ, Kennerdell JS, et al: Dysthyroid and myasthenic myopathy of the medial rectus: a clinical pathologic report. Neurology 1980; 30:939-944.

Steele JC, Richardson JC, Olsewski J: Progressive supranuclear palsy. Arch Neurol 1964; 10:333-359.

Thompson HS, Van Allen MW, von Noorden GK: The pupil in myotonic dystrophy. Invest Ophthalmol 1964; 3:325-338.

Fifth Nerve (Trigeminal) Syndromes

A. Anatomic considerations (Fig. 12-1)

1. The trigeminal nerve supplies sensation to the face via its three main branches
   V^1—Ophthalmic nerve
   V^2—Maxillary nerve
   V^3—Mandibular nerve
2. The mandibular nerve (V^3) is a motor branch to the muscles of mastication; temporalis, pterygoids, masseter

B. Oculo-facial hypesthesia

1. Look for somatotopic distribution corresponding to the three divisions of V nerve
2. Such somatotopic hypesthesia (e.g. V^1 only, or V^2 and V^3 with sparing of V^1) suggests that the lesion is more likely to be in the middle cranial fossa (cavernous sinus) or orbit, although somatotopic hypesthesia has been reported

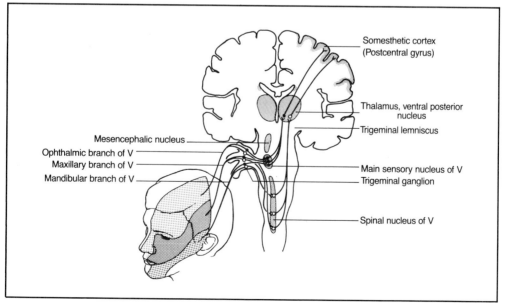

Fig. 12-1. Diagram of central pathways and peripheral innervation of the fifth nerve.

with brainstem lesions
3. Differential diagnosis of diminished sensation in the trigeminal distribution*
   a. Corneal
      1) Herpes simplex
      2) Ocular surgery
      3) Cerebellopontine angle tumors
      4) Dysautonomia
      5) Congenital
   b. Ophthalmic Division
      1) Neoplasm, orbital apex
      2) Neoplasm, superior orbital fissure
      3) Neoplasm, cavernous sinus
      4) Neoplasm, middle fossa
      5) Aneurysm, cavernous sinus
   c. Maxillary Division
      1) Orbit floor fracture
      2) Maxillary antrum carcinoma
   d. Mandibular Division
      1) Nasopharyngeal tumor
      2) Middle fossa tumor
   e. All Divisions
      1) Nasopharyngeal carcinoma
      2) Cerebellopontine angle tumors
      3) Brainstem lesions (dissociated sensory loss)
      4) Intracavernous aneurysm
      5) Demyelinative
      6) Middle fossa or Meckel's cave tumor
      7) Benign sensory neuropathy
      8) Tentorial meningioma
      9) Toxins (eg, trichlorethylene)
      10) Trigeminal neurofibroma

C. Oculo-facial pain
1. Differential diagnosis of relatively common entities associated with ocular and facial pain*
   a. Ocular
      1) Local corneal, lid and anterior segment disease
      2) Ocular inflammation
      3) Nonspecific aches, stabs and jabs
      4) Chronic ocular hypoxia, carotid occlusive disease
   b. Ophthalmic Division
      1) Migraine
      2) Raeder's paratrigeminal neuralgia
      3) Painful ophthalmoplegia syndromes

* *From Glaser JS: Neuro-ophthalmology, in Duane TD (ed.): Clinical Ophthalmology. Hagerstown, Harper & Row, 1978, Chapter 2.*

          4) Herpes zoster

          5) Referred (dural) pain, including occipital infarction

          6) Tic douloureux (infrequent in V^1)

          7) Sinusitis

    c. Maxillary Division

          1) Tic douloureux

          2) Nasopharyngeal carcinoma

          3) Temporomandibular syndrome

          4) Dental disease

          5) Sinusitis

    d. Mandibular Division

          1) Tic douloureux

          2) Dental disease

    e. Miscellaneous

          1) Atypical facial neuralgias

          2) Pain with medullary lesions

2. Specific trigeminal syndromes

    a. Referred pain

          1) Any intracranial process irritating the dural sensory fibers, which may be supplied by recurrent branches of V nerve

          2) Neck pain, e.g. from osteoarthritis in the cervical spine, may be referred to the eye because of the cervical sensory fibers traveling with the trigeminal fibers of the spinal tract of V, which extends to C-2 level

    b. Trigeminal neuralgia (Tic Douloureaux)

          1) Paroxysmal pain in the distribution of one or more of the divisions of V ($V^3 > V^2 > V^1$)

          2) Recurring, lancinating, "lightning" hemifacial pain lasting 20-30 seconds

          3) Pain may be so intense that the facial muscles contract and distort the face during an attack

          4) Frequently "triggered" by touching certain areas of the face or scalp; asymptomatic or mild headache between episodes

          5) No neurologic deficits (including normal corneal reflex)

          6) Neuralgia of more persistent nature and associated with neurologic deficits may resolve from compressive, demyelinative, or inflammatory lesion of the V nerve

    c. Herpetic neuralgia

          1) Pain of herpes zoster is described as severe, burning, aching in quality

          2) Pain occurs over distribution of a dermatome or cranial nerve, usually V^1, although it may involve the facial nerve (external ear) with ipsilateral facial palsy (Ramsay-Hunt syndrome)

          3) Pain often preceeds onset of typical rash by 4-7 days

          4) Pain usually regresses within one to two weeks, but may persist for

months or years: post-herpetic neuralgia

5) Patients typically describe dysesthesias: "crawling" and "prickly" sensations are common

d. Raeder's paratrigeminal neuralgia

1) V nerve distribution pain with ipsilateral Horner's syndrome

2) Almost exclusively in middle-aged or elderly male patients

3) May be caused by migranous dilation of the internal carotid artery with compression of the V nerve and sympathetic plexus in the middle cranial fossa

4) If the pain is persistent (not of migranous episodic nature) or if associated with cranial nerve palsy, then suspect a middle fossa tumor, aneurysm, or internal carotid artery dissection

Bibliography

BOOKS

Hasgler R, Waler AE (eds): Trigeminal neuralgia: pathogenesis and pathophysiology. Stuttgart, George Thieme Verlag, 1970.

CHAPTERS

Glaser JS: Neuro-ophthalmology, in Duane TD (ed.): Clinical Ophthalmology. Hagerstown, Harper & Row, 1978, Vol. 2, Chapter 2.

Miller NS: Walsh and Hoyt's Clinical Neuro-ophthalmology. Baltimore, Williams & Wilkins, 1985, Chapters 39-42, pp. 999-1106.

ARTICLES

Dalessio DJ: Treatment of trigeminal neuralgia. JAMA 1981; 245:2519-2520.

Davis RH, Daroff RB, Hoyt WF: Hemicrania, oculosympathetic paresis, and subcranial carotid aneurysm: Raeder's paratrigeminal syndrome (Group 2). J Neurosurg 1968; 29:94-96.

Feindel W, Penfield W, McNaughton F: The tentorial nerves and localization of intracranial pain in man. Neurology 1960; 10:555-563.

Grimson BS, Thompson HS: Raeder's syndrome: a clinical review. Surv Ophthalmol 1980; 24:199-210.

Schott GD: Neurogenic facial pain. Trans Ophthalmol Soc UK: 1980; 100:253-256.

Smith JL: Raeder's paratrigeminal syndrome. Am J Ophthalmol 1958; 46:194-201.

13

The Seven Syndromes of the Seventh (Facial) Nerve

A. Anatomic considerations

Figure 13-1 is a schematic representation of the course of the supranuclear and infranuclear fibers controlling the facial musculatures; the fibers are accompanied by the nervus intermedius (tearing, salivation, taste) as well as sensory fibers from the external ear and the nerve to the stapedius muscle; the nerve leaves the pons and travels with the eighth cranial nerve through the internal auditory canal leaving the canal through the fallopian canal, which courses inferiorly through the petrous bone, exiting through the stylomastoid foramen

B. The seven syndromes of the seventh nerve

1. Supranuclear facial palsy: results in contralateral weakness of the lower two-thirds of the face, with some weakness of the orbicularis oculi, but not as severe as with peripheral seventh nerve palsy (Fig. 13-2, A & B); does not usually require tarsorraphy
2. Cerebellopontine angle tumor
   a. Total ipsilateral facial weakness
   b. Decreased tearing (nervus intermedius)
   c. Hyperacusis (nerve to stapedius muscle)
   d. Decreased taste of anterior two-thirds of tongue (nervus intermedius and chorda tympani)
   e. Associated neurologic deficits: V, VI, VIII, Horner's syndrome, gaze palsy, nystagmus, papilledema, cerebellar dysfunction
3. Geniculate ganglionitis (Ramsay-Hunt syndrome, zoster oticus)
   a. Same findings as (2) except no associated neurologic deficits except for possibly a VIII nerve involvement
   b. May see zoster vesicles on tympanic membrane, in external auditory canal, or on external ear
4. Isolated ipsilateral tear deficiency
   a. Nasopharyngeal carcinoma may affect the vidian nerve or spheno-palatine ganglion; often accompanying sixth nerve palsy due to cavernous sinus involvement

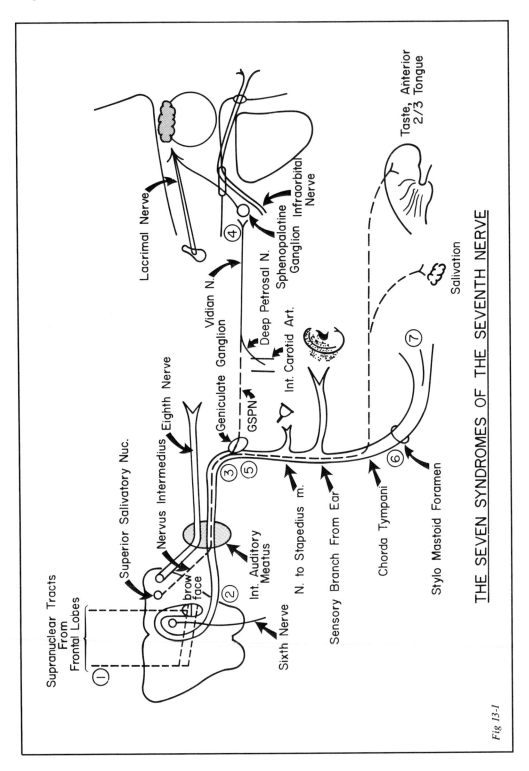

Fig 13-1

THE SEVEN SYNDROMES OF THE SEVENTH NERVE

5. Bell's palsy
   a. Common idiopathic facial palsy, possibly due to edema of VII nerve within fallopian canal
   b. Same findings as (2) except for no associated neurologic deficits; tearing may be normal
   c. Complete recovery, with 60 days in 75% of patients; with steroid therapy, recovery over 90%
6. Isolated total ipsilateral facial palsy
   a. Mastoidopathy, facial trauma, parotid gland surgery
7. Isolated partial ipsilaterial facial palsy
   a. Only certain branches of VII nerve are affected

C. Facial diplegia
   1. Brainstem contusion
   2. Brainstem stroke (basilar artery)
   3. Brainstem glioma
   4. Moebius syndrome: aplasia of VII nerve nuclei in brainstem; often accompanied by
      a. Bilateral VI nerve palsies
      b. Palatal and lingual palsy
      c. Deafness
      d. Deficiencies of pectoral and lingual muscles
      e. Extremity defects: syndactyly, supernumary digits, absent finges, toes
   5. Myasthenia gravis

D. Crocodile tears (Gustolacrimal reflex)
   1. Any patient with VII palsy which has affected the fibers stimulating tearing and salivation may experience tearing at mealtime due to aberrant regeneration or misdirection of fibers, so that when neural stimulus for salivation is transmitted, it results in stimulation of tearing

E. Spastic paretic facial contracture
   1. Unilateral spastic facial contracture with associated facial weakness
   2. Indicative of intrinsic pontine neoplasm
   3. Due to damage of VII n. nucleus (facial paresis) and its supranuclear connections (facial spasticity)

F. Blepharospasm
   1. Bilateral, episodic, involuntary contractions of the orbicularis oculi
   2. At times associated with involuntary spasm of the lower facial musculature: orofacial dyskenesia or Meige syndrome
   3. Etiology unkown
   4. Treatment
      a. pharmacologic: Clonopin
      b. chemodenervation: botulinum toxin
      c. surgery: selective VII n. sectioning

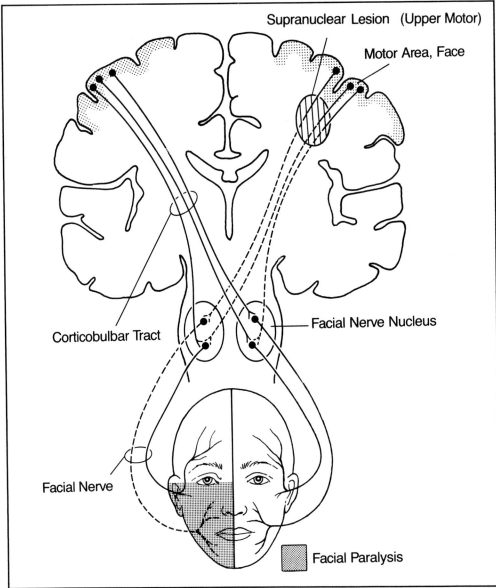

Fig. 13-2A. Facial weakness due to upper motor neuron lesion.

G. Hemifacial spasm
1. Unilateral spasm involving half of facial muscles, typically lasting several minutes at a time
2. Painless, no sensory loss
3. Etiology: aberrant vascular loop compressing VII n. in subarachnoid space where it exits the pons
4. Treatment
   a. pharmacologic: carbamazepine (Tegretol)
   b. chemodenervation: botulinum toxin

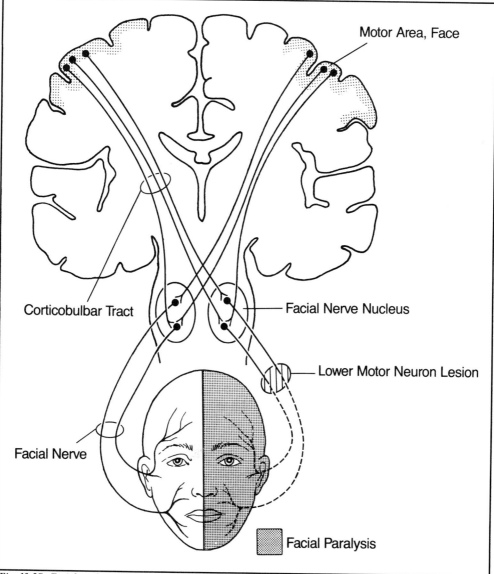

Fig. 13-2B. Facial weakness due to lower motor neuron lesion.

    c. surgery: posterior fossa craniotomy with insertion of inert material between vascular loop and VII n

H. Facial myokymia
  1. Usually benign, self-limited
  2. If persistent over weeks or months then consider
    a. Multiple sclerosis
    b. Brainstem glioma
    c. Brainstem stroke

Bibliography

CHAPTERS

Miller NR: Walsh and Hoyt's Clinical Neuro-Ophthalmogy. Baltimore, Williams & Wilkins, 1985, Chapter 38, pp. 932-995.

ARTICLES

Frueh DR, Felt DP, Wojno JH, et al: Treatment of blepharospasm with botulinum toxim. Arch Ophthalmol 1984; 102:1464-1468.

Gillum WN, Anderson RL: Blepharospasm surgery: an anatomical approach. Arch Ophthalmol 1981; 99:1056-1062.

Jankovic J, Havins WE, Wilkins RB: Blinking and blepharospasm: mechanics, diagnosis and management. JAMA 1982; 248:3160-3164.

Jannetta PJ: The cause of hemifacial spasm: definitive microsurgical treatment at the brainstem in 31 patients. Trans Am Acad Ophthalmol Otolaryngol 1974; 80:319-322.

Scott AB: Botulinum toxin injection of eye muscles to correct strabismus. Trans Am Ophthalmol Soc 1981; 79:734-700.

Sogg RL, Hoyt WF, Boldrey E: Spastic paretic facial contraction: a rare sign of brain stem tumor. Neurology 1963; 13:607-612.

Towfighi J, Marks K, Palmer E, et al: Möbius syndrome: neuro-pathologic observations. Acta Neuropathol 1979; 48:11-17.

Headache

Patrick S. O'Connor, M.D.

A. Anatomic considerations
  1. Pain sensitive structures within the cranium include
     a. Great venous sinuses and tributaries
     b. Parts of dura at base of skull
     c. Dural and cerebral arteries at base of brain
  2. Six basic courses of intracranial headache
     a. Traction on tributary veins or displacement of great venous sinuses
     b. Traction on middle meningeal arteries
     c. Traction on large cerebral arteries or branches at the base
     d. Distension and dilation of intracranial arteries
     e. Inflammation of pain sensitive structures
     f. Direct pressure on cranial or cervical nerves (fifth nerve above tentorium and ninth, tenth, eleventh, and twelfth and upper cervical below tentorium)
  3. Extracranial sources of head pain include
     a. Fasciae, muscles and galea
     b. Extracranial arteries and veins of the head and neck
     c. Mucous membranes, tympanic membrane, etc.

B. History is the key to diagnosis (95% of headache patients have a normal examination)
  1. Where?
  2. How long?
  3. How often?
  4. Characteristics of pain (what makes it better or worse)
  5. Accompanying signs and symptoms

C. Headache Syndromes
  1. Muscle contraction (tension-anxiety headache)
     a. Account of 90% of all headaches
     b. Acute contraction headache
        1) Emotional or physical stress
        2) Sustained contraction of neck and scalp muscles
        3) Pain usually dull and non throbbing (tenderness and knotting noted in

            strap muscles of neck)

          4) Can be superimposed on many other headache types

    c. Chronic muscle contraction headache

          1) Symptoms of band around head, tightness, head in a vise

          2) Depression common denominator in these chronic, long standing headaches

2. Migraine

    a. Migraine is a common neurologic disorder said to affect 15-19% of men and 25-29% of women. Headache is never the sole manifestation of migraine nor indeed a necessary feature of migraine attacks. It can occur at any age, a strong family history is common as well as a history of car sickness in childhood. Frequently, erroneously attributed by the patient to "sinus" disease

    b. Classic migraine

          1) Sharply defined aura, usually visual, lasting 20-40 minutes

          2) Throbbing pain which is usually unilateral

          3) Anorexia, nausea, noise and light sensitivity frequently accompany headache

          4) Other nonvisual symptoms such as hemiparesis, dysphasia, and cloudy thinking may proceed the headache

          5) Strong family history 80% of the time

          6) Only 20% of migraineurs have classic migraine

    c. Common migraine

          1) Prodrome not well defined, may proceed headache by hours or days and includes mood disorders, GI distress, fatigue

          2) Photophobia, nausea and/or vomiting and anorexia a common finding

          3) Ocular symptoms include conjunctival injection and tearing, no visual aura

    d. Complicated migraine: paroxysmal neurologic deficits that occur beyond headache phase, usually transient but may be permanent

          1) Cerebral migraine: include motor, visual or other sensory deficits

              a) Hemiplegic migraine—partial or total hemiparesis or hemiplegia (may be familial)

              b) Transient and rarely permanent homonomous or quadrantic visual field defects

              c) Speech disorders

              d) Except for familial hemiplegic migraine, all patients with hemiparesis should be evaluated for a structural lesion by CT scanning

          2) Ophthalmoplegic migraine

              a) Onset usually before age 10

              b) Third nerve affected 10 to 1 over sixth

              c) Pupil and accommodation frequently involved

              d) Ophthalmoplegia occurs at height of headache persisting when headache clears (may last days to weeks)

              e) Strict criteria for diagnosis

1. Onset first decade
2. History of typical migraine
3. Ophthalmoplegia ipsilateral to headache
4. Negative cranial CT scanning
5. Some believe negative angiography also necessary

3) Basilar artery migraine (Bickerstaff's migraine)
   a) Mimics vertebrobasilar insufficiency seen in elderly patients
   b) Distinguished by severe headache and vomiting following onset
   c) Usually affects young women with strong family history of migraine
   d) Neurologic symptoms usually clear but permanent deficits can occur

4) Cluster headache (Horton's headache, histamine cephalgia)
   a) Typically awakens patient early in the morning
   b) Severe pain in the distribution of the external carotid (frontal or frontotemporal pain)
   c) Headache accompanied by ipsilateral Horner's syndrome, lacrimation and rhinorrhea
   d) Occasional conjunctival edema and injection
   e) Occurs in third and fourth decade with 5 to 1 male predominance
   f) Patient tends to pace floor until the pain subsides in thirty minutes to three to four hours
   g) Post-ganglionic Horner's persists in 10% of patients

5) Raeder's syndrome (painful Horner's with pain usually in V^1 distribution)
   a) Found in middle aged or elderly males
   b) May be caused by migrainous dilation of the internal carotid artery with compression of V and sympathetic plexis in the middle cranial fossa
   c) Two types
      1. Type one: other cranial nerves involved. Requires complete neuroradiographic investigation to rule out a parasellar mass
      2. Type two: pain in ophthalmic division with post-ganglionic Horner's only. Pain may last days to weeks or months. This type can also rarely occur with fibromuscular dysplasia or spontaneous carotid dissection

6) Retinal migraine: transient and occasionally permanent monocular visual disturbance occurring in a young person with a strong history of migraine
   a) Headache frequently absent during spell
   b) When no previous headache history must rule out embolic and vasculopathic disease, optic disc infarctions have also been reported

7) Migraine equivalent or variant
   a) Denotes symptomatology believed to be migrainous in nature, due

to presumed cerebral ischemia with spreading depression including cyclic vomiting, nausea, abdominal pain or motion sickness in children as well as periodic fever and mood changes in children and adults

8) Acephalgic migraine (migraine without a headache) denotes the occurrence of neurologic symptoms usually associated with migraine but without a headache phase

    a) Visual symptoms include scintillating scotomas, transient hemianopia, amaurosis fugax, altitudinal field loss, tunnel vision, and diplopia

    b) Other neurologic symptoms and signs frequently noted

    c) Positive family history of migraine occurs in only 24% of these patients

    d) Can present at any age, frequently confused with transient cerebral attacks when it occurs in patients over the age of 40

    e) Diagnosis of acephalgic migraine can be made when the typical march of scintillating scotomas or other neurologic accompaniments of migraine is present. If this march is present no further evaluation is necessary; if march absent the diagnosis is one of exclusion. This is one of the most common forms of migraine seen by the ophthalmologist

3. Headache associated with brain tumor or other intracranial disease

  a. Usually appears quite suddenly

  b. May be mild or intermittent initially but progressively worsens

  c. May be worse in head down position, coughing, straining

  d. Other symptoms usually present

4. Other causes

  a. Hypertension should always be a diagnostic consideration

  b. Sinus disease

    1) Dull, aching, and constant pain the tenderness almost universally found over the involved sinus

    2) Headaches usually aggravated by change in atmospheric pressure

    3) Many patients call migraine headaches "sinus"

  c. Headache may also be associated with temporomandibular joint dysfunction, fever, raised intracranial pressure; and ocular inflammation

  d. Headache rarely due to "eyestrain" but when due to asthenopia, pain is precipitated by eye use and relieved by rest

  e. Other causes of headache include conversion reaction, herpetic disease and greater occipital neuralgia

Bibliography

BOOKS

Dalessio DJ (ed): Wolff's headache and other head pain. New York, Oxford University Press, 1980.

Sacks OW: Migraine, the evolution of a common disorder. Los Angeles, University of California Press, 1970.

CHAPTERS

Miller NR: Walsh and Hoyt's Clinical Neuro-Ophthalmology. Baltimore, Williams & Wilkins, 1985, Chapter 43, pp. 1107-1121.

Troost BT: Migraine, In Duane TD (ed.): Clinical Ophthalmology. Hagerstown, Harper & Row, 1978, Vol. 2, Chapter 19.

ARTICLES

Bickerstaff ER: Basilar artery migraine. Lancet 1961; 1:15-17.

Bode DD, Jr: Ocular pain secondary to occipital neuritis. Ann Ophthalmol 1979; 11:589-594.

Carroll D: Retinal migraine. Headache 1970; 10:9-13.

David RH, Daroff RB, Hoyt WF: Hemicrania, oculosympathetic paresis, and subcranial carotid aneurysm: Raeder's paratrigeminal syndrome (Group 2). J Neurosurg 1968; 29:94-96.

Fisher CM: Late-life migraine accompaniments as a cause of unexplained transient ischemic attacks. Can J Neurol Sci 1980; 7:9-17.

Friedman AP, Harter DH, Merritt HH: Ophthalmoplegic migraine. Arch eurol 1962; 7:320-327.

Goldor H: Headache and eye pain. In Gay AJ, Burde RM (eds): Clinical concepts in neuro-ophthalmology. Int Ophthalmol Clin 1967; 7(4):697-705.

O'Connor PS, Tredici TJ: Acephalgic migraine. Fifteen years experience. Ophthalmology 1981; 88:999-1003.

O'Hara M, O'Connor PS: Migrainous optic neuropathy. J Clin Neuro-ophthalmol 1984; 4:85-90.

Riley FC, Moyer MJ: Oculosympathetic paresis associated with cluster headaches. Am J Ophthalmol 1971; 72:763-768.

Spector RH: Migraine. Surv Ophthalmol 1984; 29:193-207.

15

Ancillary Clinical Procedures

Patrick S. O'Connor, M.D.

A. Superficial Temporal Artery Biopsy

The temporal artery is a terminal branch of the external carotid artery. Because of its ready accessibility and high frequency of involvement in giant cell arteritis, it is most often biopsied to establish the diagnosis

1. The artery lies in front of the ear over the zygomatic process of the temporal bone. It divides into a posterior parietal branch and anterior frontal branch (Fig. 15-1A). The frontal branch lies above the temporalis fascia and follows a tortuous course across the forehead to an anastomosis with the supraorbital and supra-trochlear branches of the ophthalmic artery

2. The frontal branch is usually chosen for biopsy. The artery classically is described as being nodular and tender when involved. However, the vessel may feel and look normal yet prove abnormal on histologic examination

3. After the frontal branch is identified the area should be prepared by shaving the overlying skin

4. The shaved area is scrubbed with Betadine solution for five minutes with 4 × 4's. The area is then dried and a sterile plastic eye drape is applied to the biopsy area

5. The vessel is carefully palpated and its course marked for four to five centimeters

6. Plain 2% xylocaine is used for local infiltration. Epinephrine should be avoided because of its vasospastic potential. Five to ten cc should be injected 1 cm to either side of the artery and parallel to but not directly over the artery itself

7. The skin incision is made with a No. 15 Bard Parker blade directly along the skin mark. Traction at each end of the incision site is used when making the full thickness incision through the skin. 4 × 4's can then be used at the incision edges to control bleeding. Rarely is cautery or ligature needed

8. Sub-cutaneous blunt dissection is done using a hemostat or small blunt-nosed scissors. Dissection with sharp instruments is never performed. The frontal branch is identified above the temporalis fascia (Fig. 15-1B)

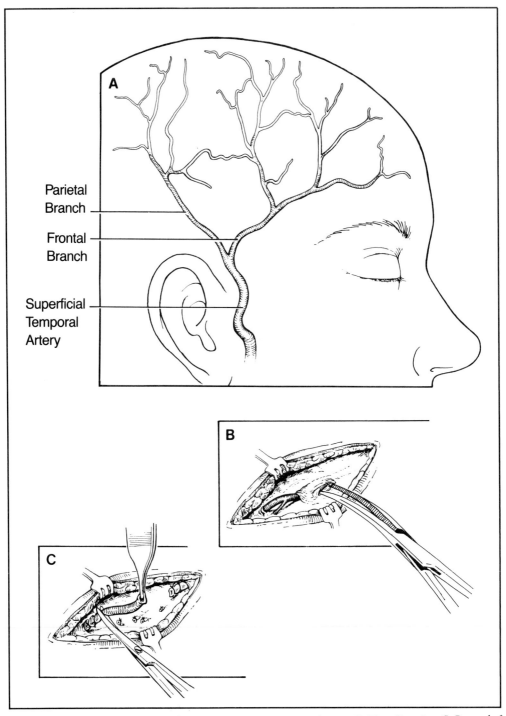

Parietal
Branch

Frontal
Branch

Superficial
Temporal
Artery

Fig. 15-1. Steps in performing superficial temporal artery biopsy. A: Localization. B: Blunt dissection. C: Removal of biopsy specimen.

9. If pulsations were obtained at the beginning of the procedure the dissection bed is repeatedly palpated to identify the course of the artery

10. If the pulse disappears, several drops of proparacaine can be instilled on the wound reducing vasospasm

11. Two 4-0 black silk sutures are passed below the artery, one proximally and one distally to permit manipulation without the use of instruments that could cause crush artifact. At least three centimeters of artery should be isolated and freed from surrounding tissue. Branches of the artery are ligated with 4-0 chromic suture. The artery is ligated as far proximally and distally as possible. Three square knots should be placed with the silk sutures and the ends not cut too closely. Some prefer a double ligature proximally and distally (Fig. 15-1C)

12. Once bleeding is controlled the wound is closed with 6-0 black silk sutures. A pressure dressing is applied for 24 hours

13. The most common late complication is hemorrhage. There is one case report of a patient with asymptomatic internal carotid occlusion who suffered a stroke during biopsy of the ipsilateral temporal artery because of interruption of collateral flow. It may be prudent to compress the vessel for several minutes to insure that critical collateral flow will not be compromised if it is removed

14. Skin sutures are removed in five days

B. The Tensilon Test

1. Tensilon (edrophonium hydrochloride) is supplied in a single dose, 10 mg/1 ml breakneck vial

2. A definite end point must be selected. If the patient has no findings at the time of examination testing should be postponed. If ptosis is present it should be documented photographically before and after injection

3. If diplopia is present careful measurement of the deviation should be carried out before, immediately after and three to four minutes following injection. Three types of responses may occur in myasthenic patients: 1) an improvement in alignment (large tropia becomes smaller); 2) a worsening of alignment (a small tropia becomes a large tropia); 3) a reversal of alignment (a left hypertropia becomes a right hypertropia). Type 1 responses occur only in myasthenics while type 2 and 3 responses may be seen in non-myasthenic ophthalmoplegics

4. Procedures in adults
   a. Tensilon should be drawn up in a 1 cc tuberculin syringe
   b. 0.4 mg of injectable atropine should also be drawn up in another 1 cc tuberculin syringe
   c. A 10 cc syringe is filled with injectable saline
   d. A scalp vein needle is placed in a dorsal arm or hand vein
   e. 1 ml of saline solution is injected and the patient observed for one minute
   f. .2 ml of Tensilon is injected and the tubing flushed with 1 ml of saline and observe for one minute
   g. If no response, a bolus of .8 ml of Tensilon is injected and the tubing flushed with another 1 ml of saline; atropine is then connected to the tubing

h. Atropine is only used with severe bradycardia, angina, bronchospasm
5. In children and uncooperative adults 0.4 mg of atropine is given intra-muscularly fifteen minutes prior to the injection of neostigmine (Prostigmin) and the dose calculated as follows: Weight (kg)/70(kg) times 1.5 mg = dose. Patient is reexamined 30 to 45 minutes after injection

C. Forced Duction Testing (Fig. 15-2)

1. In patients with acquired diplopia and an incomitant deviation, forced duction testing can eliminate the need for extensive neurologic investigation if restriction is found. Remember many patients with thyroid myopathy have only subtle or no other signs of classic thyroid eye disease
2. Three drops of topical proparacaine solution are instilled in the inferior cul de sac of each eye. During this time a cotton-tipped applicator is soaked with similar solution
3. The patient is asked to look in the direction of gaze limitation. The cotton-tipped applicator is placed on the conjunctiva anterior to the presumed restricted muscle
4. The conjunctiva is grasped with toothed forceps and the globe passively rotated in the direction of the limited duction
5. The same procedure is carried out in the fellow eye and the relative limitation compared. In subtle cases, repeated comparisons between the two eyes may be necessary
6. At times with attempted forced ductions the globe is displaced backward into the orbit. This phenomenon must be observed, or the examiner may believe the eye moves more easily than it actually does
7. Occasionally patients are not able to cooperate for forced duction testing. In these cases measurement of the intra-ocular pressure in the primary position and again with the eyes moved into the direction of limited gaze is compared. A pressure rise of greater than 4 mm in moving from one gaze position to another is felt to be diagnostic of a restrictive process

D. Confrontation Visual Fields

1. Many significant neurologic field defects can be found with simple confrontation techniques
2. The best technique of finger counting fields evaluates both sides of the vertical meridian with care taken not to move the fingers in various quadrants since many patients with a damaged occipital lobe can still appreciate motion in the blind field (Riddoch phenomenon)
3. Procedure (Fig. 15-3)
   a. One eye of the patient is occluded
   b. The patient is then asked to look at the examiner's nose maintaining steady fixation. The test distance should be approximately one meter between patient and examiner
   c. Finger counting is then carried out in the four quadrants; superior temporal, inferior temporal, inferior nasal, and superior nasal. Between one and five fingers is presented and the number varied. The fingers are presented in a static fashion 20 and 30 degrees from fixation

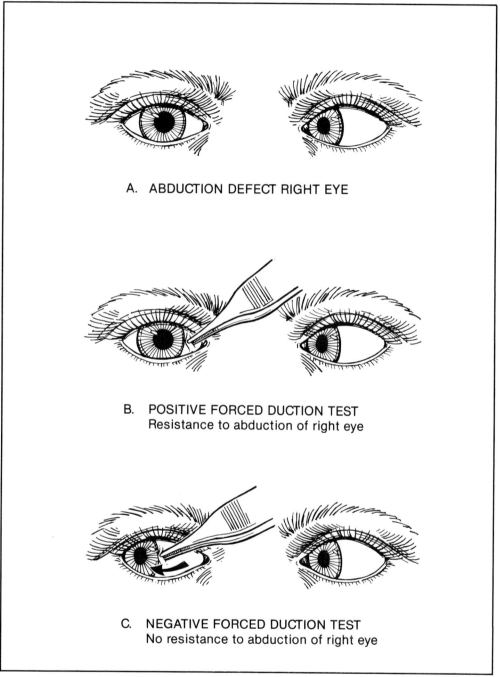

A. ABDUCTION DEFECT RIGHT EYE

B. POSITIVE FORCED DUCTION TEST
Resistance to abduction of right eye

C. NEGATIVE FORCED DUCTION TEST
No resistance to abduction of right eye

Fig. 15-2. Forced duction testing.

167

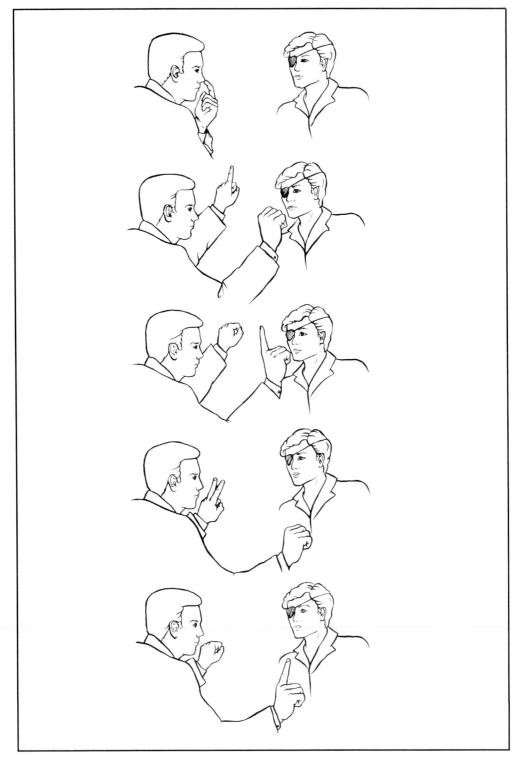

Fig. 15-3. Confrontation visual field technique.

    d. Double simultaneous stimulation. The same number of fingers are simultaneously presented on each side of the vertical meridian with careful monitoring of the patient's fixation. Parietal lobe lesions can result in visual field inattention to simultaneous targets even when individually presented targets can be identified

    e. Hemifield comparison. Again with controlled fixation, both hands are held on either side of the vertical meridian and the patient is asked to compare their appearance (i.e. one "clearer" or "darker" than the other). The patient is always asked to point to the abnormal hand to reduce confusion. If for example the hand in the patient's temporal field appears dimmer then both hands are again presented in the temporal field above and below the horizontal and the patient asked to identify the clearer of the two allowing definition of whether the defect is denser above or below

    f. The same procedure is carried out in the other eye

4. Finger counting fields should be performed as part of every routine examination not just in patients suspected of having neurologic disease

5. A great deal of information can also be gained from subjective visual fields in which the patient covers one eye and focuses on the center of the examiner's face usually the nose. The patient is then asked if he can see both ears simultaneously, the head and the chin, the examiner's shoulder, tie, etc. Frequently, scotomas not easily identified on perimetry are recognized as a central dimming by the patient when viewing the examiner's face. The same is also true for early inferior altitudinal defects which may be subtle on perimetry but easily identified by the patient on subjective examination

Bibliography

CHAPTERS

Anderson DR: Testing the field of vision. St. Louis, CV Mosby, 1975, Chapter 19, pp. 228-249.

Burde RM, Savino PJ, Trobe JD: Clinical decisions in neuro-ophthalmology. St. Louis, CV Mosby, 1985, Chapter 5, pp. 147-195.

ARTICLES

Alestig K, Barr J: Giant cell arteritis. Lancet 1963; 1:1228-1230.

Brennan J, McCrary JA: Diagnosis of superficial temporal arteritis. Ann Ophthalmol 1975; 7:1125-1129.

Fisher CM: Giant cell arteritis: discussion. Trans Am Neurol Ass 1971; 96:12-15.

Gamblin GT, Harper DG, Galentine P, et al: Prevalence of increased intraocular pressure in Grave's disease: evidence of frequent subclinical ophthalmology. N Engl J Med 1983; 308:420-424.

Keltner JL: Giant-cell arteritis. Ophthalmology 1982; 89:1101-1110.

Simmons RJ, Cogan DG: Occult temporal arteritis. Arch Ophthalmol 1962; 68:8-18.

Trobe JD, Acosta PC, Krischer JP, et al: Confrontation visual field techniques in the detection of anterior visual pathway lesions. Ann Neurol 1981; 10:28-34.

Zappia RJ, Winkleman JZ, Gay AJ: Intraocular pressure changes in normal subjects and the adhesive muscle syndrome. Am J Ophthalmol 1971; 71:880-883.

Index